Makin' It Healthy
Recipes

Geetu Makin

Copyright

Hardcover: 979-8-9928765-3-6

Copyright @2025 by Geetu Makin

All rights reserved.

No portion of this book may be reproduced in any form without written permission from the publisher or author, except as permitted by U.S. copyright law.

No AI Training: Use of this publication—including its text, photographs, or artwork—for the purpose of training generative artificial intelligence ("AI") technologies is expressly prohibited, without limiting the author's (and publisher's) exclusive rights under copyright law.

Editor: Michelle Emmanuelli

Photographer: Michael Thompson

Other Photo Credit: Farah Ghazal

Cover & Interior Design: Heisy Amil

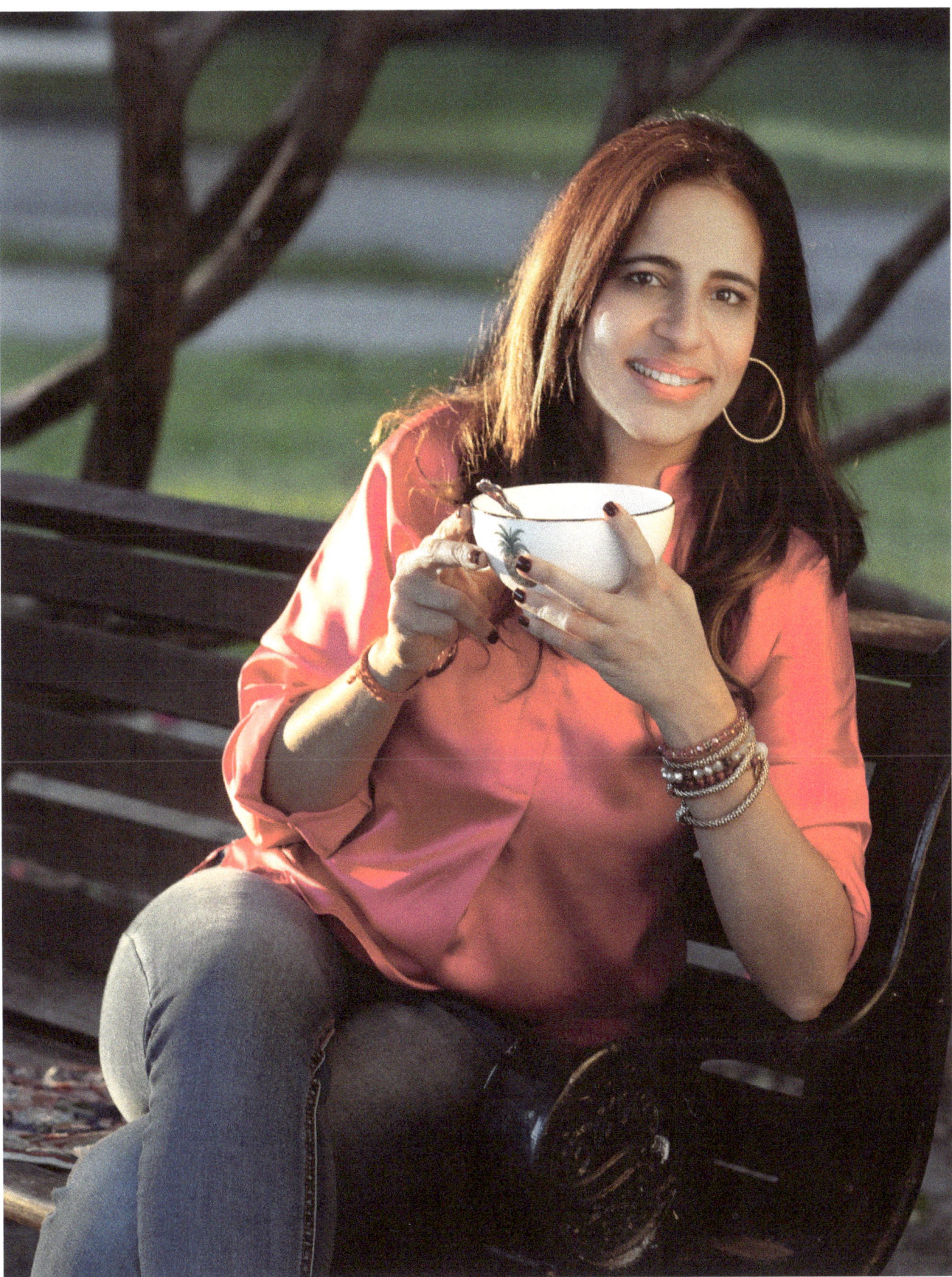

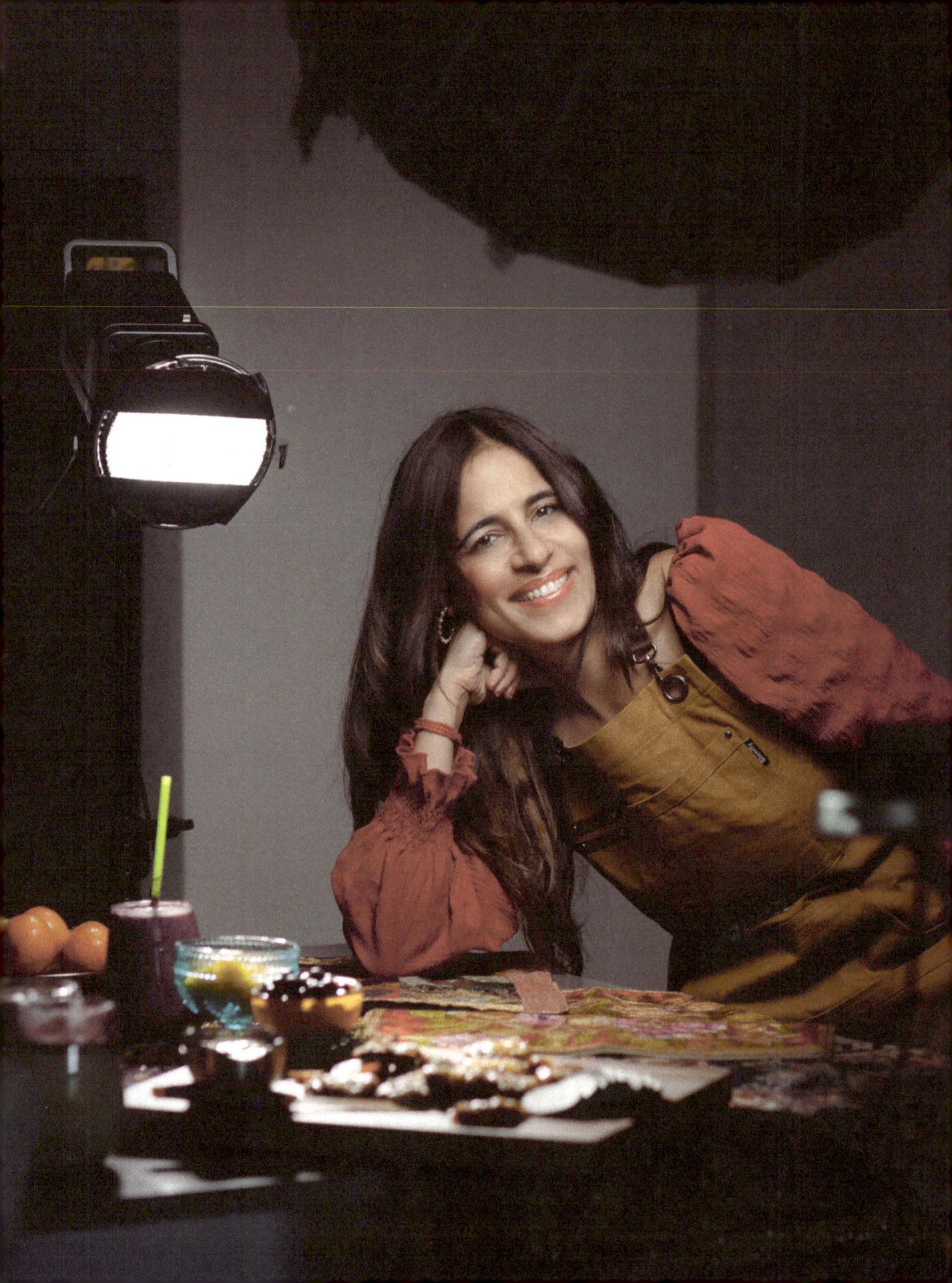

table of contents

dedication	7
introduction	9
family-friendly nourishing recipes for adults & teenagers	12
• the ultimate creamy butter chicken	15
• balanced chicken biryani feast	23
• 7-lentil harmony curry soup	29
• chickpea curry salad	37
• malai chicken kebab with herb-infused white sauce	45
• crispy aloo tikki with mint chutney	53
• fresh start mint chutney	59
• spinach paneer bliss curry	65
• wrap-tastic paneer kathi roll	71
• protein-packed mediterranean bean delight	77
• palak infused chicken	83
• gobi aloo power bowl	89
• kheerlicious	95
kid-friendly nutrient fueled favorites	100
• rainbow grilled cheese sandwich	103
• oatfully yours baked donuts	109
• almond glow baked donuts	115
• rainbow smoothies: a colorful adventure in every sip	121
• berry sunrise smoothie	126
• mango oat dream smoothie	129
• oatmazing berry blend smoothie	130
• mini zucchini veggie power pizzas	133
• banana sushi bites	139
acknowledgements	145

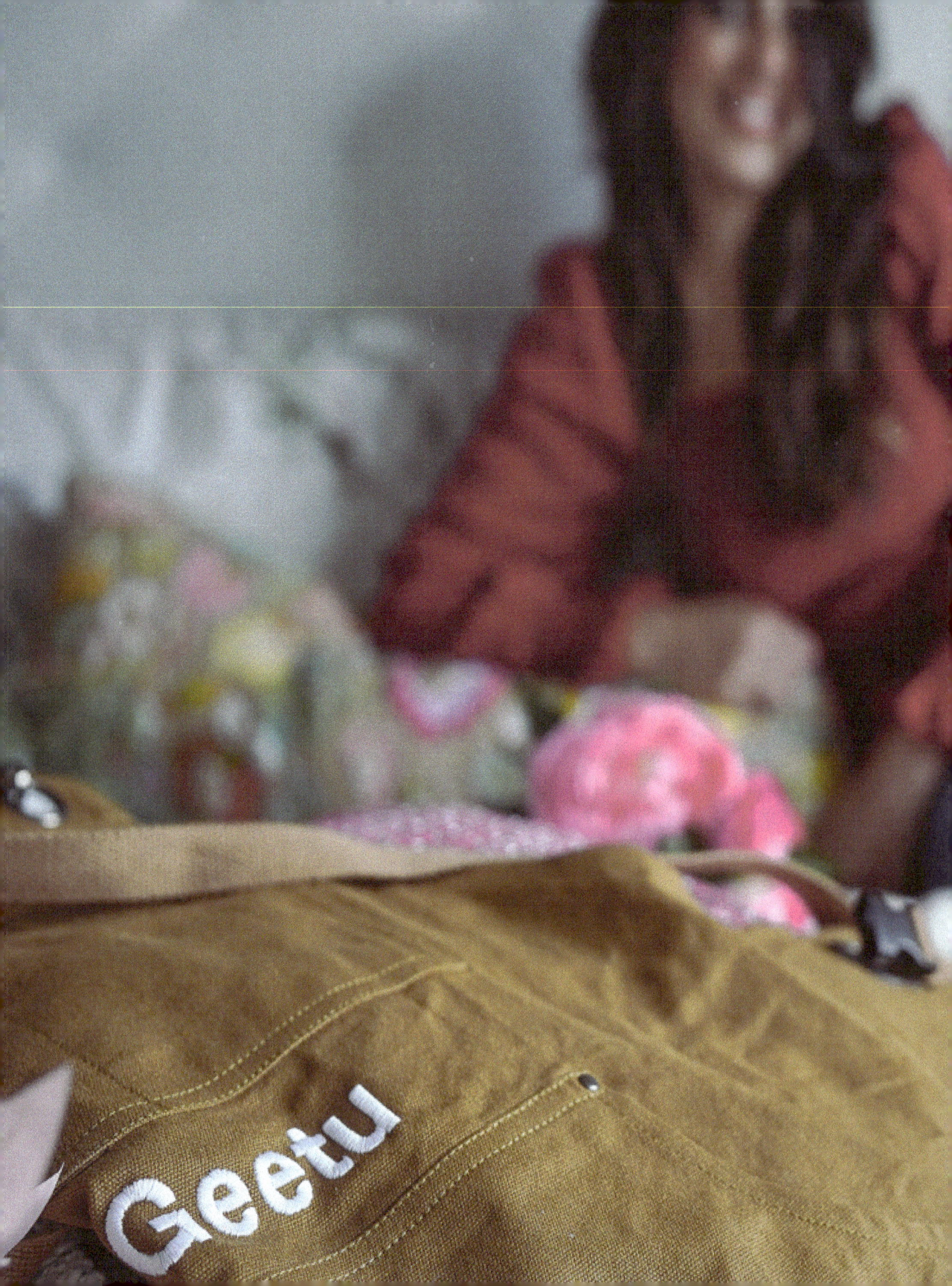

For My Mom

The heart behind every recipe

This book is for the woman who first sparked my love for cooking.

Mom, your warmth, your wisdom, and your belief in nourishing food shaped who I am and how I cook today.

This cookbook is a piece of my heart—and you're at the center of it. From rolling rotis by your side to tasting dal straight from the pot, you filled our home with flavors I still carry with me.

In the aroma of cumin and the rhythm of chopping herbs, I hear your voice.

You taught me that food could heal, connect, and tell stories—and that nourishment starts with care. Every page in this book carries a piece of what you taught me—with love, with flavor, and always with heart.

You were the recipe I followed before I knew how to cook.

Xoxo

Geetu

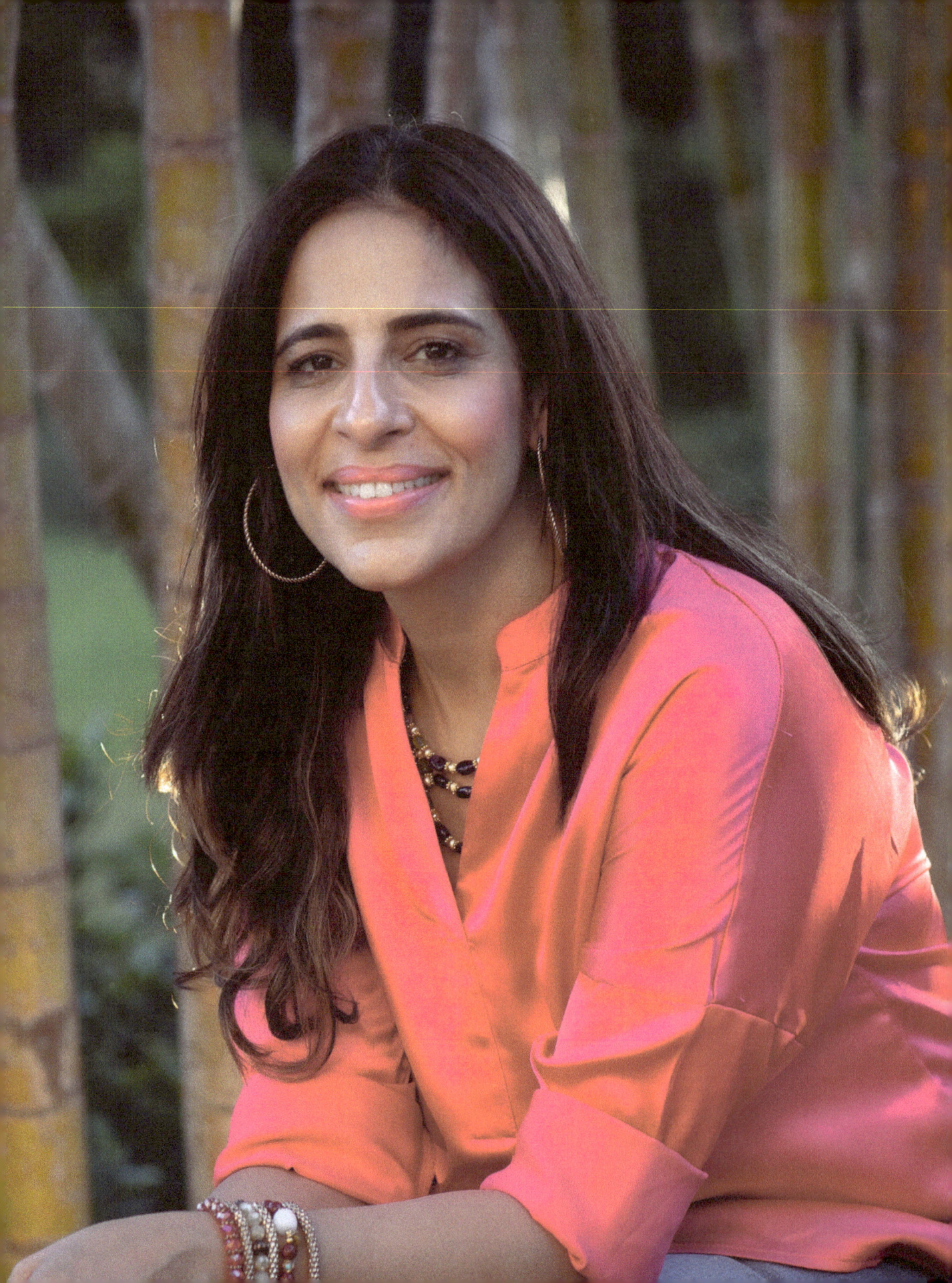

introduction

My Journey into the World of Nutrition

Healthy eating has always been close to my heart, but my journey into nutrition started long before I fully understood its impact. Growing up, my home was always filled with the comforting aromas of wholesome, home-cooked meals, all thanks to my mom. She taught me that food wasn't just about filling our bellies but about nourishing our bodies and souls, creating memories, and embracing balance. Those early experiences planted the seed for my passion for cooking and nutrition. From a young age, I developed a deep appreciation for fresh, natural ingredients and their incredible ability to nourish and energize us.

As I grew older, I became increasingly aware of how food directly impacts our health, energy, and well-being. I noticed that what we eat can either make us feel vibrant or leave us feeling sluggish. This realization sparked my interest in understanding nutrition more deeply. I began experimenting with different ingredients, learning how to balance flavors and textures in healthy, delicious ways. The more I explored, the more I realized that healthy eating isn't about restriction or deprivation, it's about making mindful choices and finding joy in nourishing meals.

My passion for healthy eating led me to pursue a formal education in nutrition, where I gained a deeper understanding of how food can heal, energize, and support us in living our best lives. Over time, I found that incorporating whole foods, reducing processed ingredients, and focusing on flavor-rich dishes was the key to making nutritious meals both satisfying and delicious.

As I advanced in my education and earned my certification in nutrition, I gained a deeper insight into how food influences our overall well-being. I learned how the right nutrients can boost energy, support digestion, and improve mental clarity. The more I studied, the more I realized that food isn't just something we eat, it sends signals to our cells and supports healing.

Food has always been more than just fuel for me—it's a way to nurture the body, mind, and soul. My journey into healthy eating wasn't always a straight path. Like many, I once struggled with understanding what "healthy" truly meant. Between fad diets, conflicting nutritional advice, and the constant hustle of life, I often found myself overwhelmed and frustrated.

But everything changed when I started focusing on whole, nourishing foods and a balanced approach to eating. I realized that healthy eating doesn't have to be bland, complicated, restrictive, or boring; it can be colorful, delicious, and truly fulfilling. Through trial and error, I discovered simple ways to make nutritious eating a sustainable and joyful part of life.

I believe that nourishing your body should feel good, taste amazing, and be something you look forward to every day.

Through this journey, I've discovered that the most effective approach to nutrition is one that is balanced, enjoyable, and designed to nourish both the body and soul sustainably.

What truly deepened my love for healthy cooking, however, was the art of pairing ingredients. I found so much joy in discovering how different foods complement one another—not just in flavor, but in how they work together to nourish and strengthen the body. From combining vitamin-rich vegetables with healthy fats for better absorption to pairing proteins and whole grains for sustained energy, every meal became an opportunity to create something both delicious and beneficial.

That's what inspired me to write this cookbook. I wanted to share the magic of food synergy—the way simple, wholesome ingredients can come together to create meals that are greater than the sum of their parts. This book reflects my passion for balanced nutrition, whole foods, and the belief that eating well should be both enjoyable and effortless.

As I continue on this journey, I am excited to share my love for healthy, flavorful cooking with others. Whether it's a smoothie packed with fruits and veggies or a spice-infused curry, I believe that food should always be a source of nourishment, joy, and connection. Healthy eating isn't just a trend, it's a way of life that can enhance our overall well-being and bring us closer to the best versions of ourselves.

This cookbook is a reflection of that journey. Inside, you'll find wholesome, delicious recipes designed to energize your body, support your well-being, and bring joy to your table. Whether you're looking for quick weekday meals, nutrient-packed snacks, or comforting dishes with a healthy twist, there's something here for everyone.

My hope is that these recipes inspire you to embrace a balanced, nourishing way of eating—one that makes you feel your absolute best, without sacrificing flavor or the love of good food.

So, grab your apron and let's create meals that nourish from the inside out—because healthy eating should be as delicious as it is nourishing!

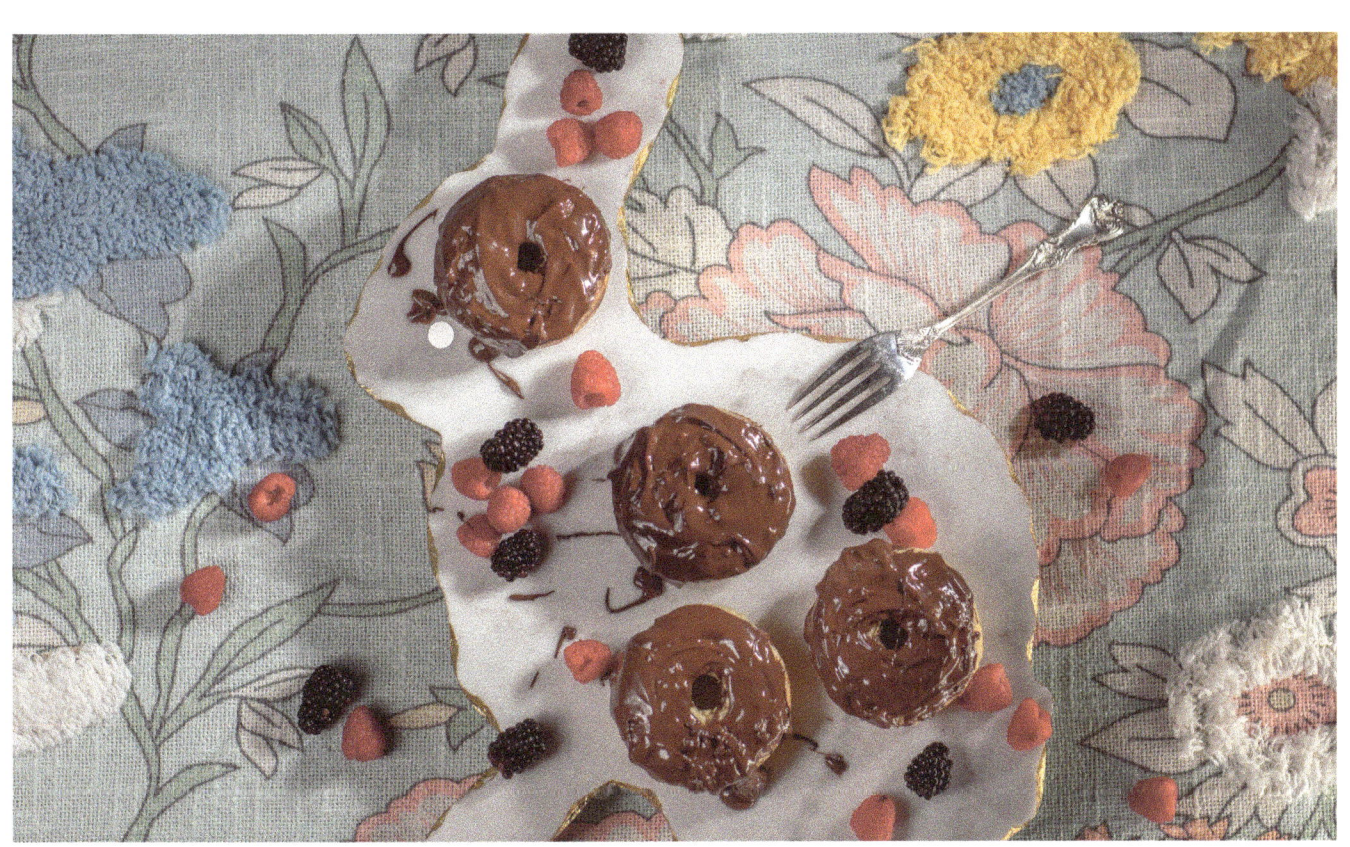

family-friendly
nourishing recipes for adults & teenagers

- the ultimate creamy butter chicken   15
- balanced chicken biryani feast   23
- 7-lentil harmony curry soup   29
- chickpea curry salad   37
- malai chicken kebab with herb-infused white sauce   45
- crispy aloo tikki with mint chutney   53
- fresh start mint chutney   59
- spinach paneer bliss curry   65
- wrap-tastic paneer kathi roll   71
- protein-packed mediterranean bean delight   77
- palak infused chicken   83
- gobi aloo power bowl   89
- kheerlicious   95

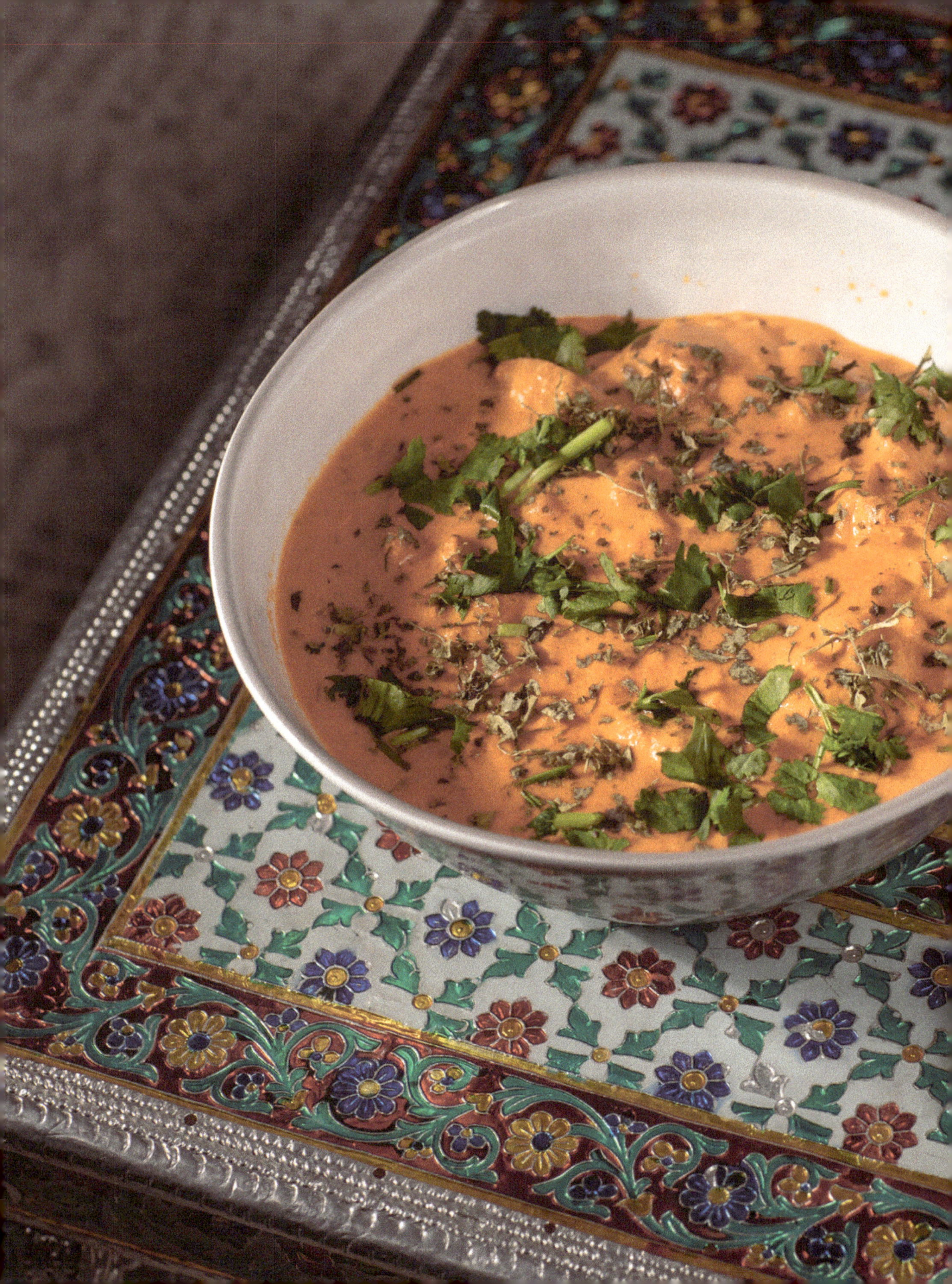

the ultimate creamy butter chicken

Food we create has the power to nourish not just our bodies, but our hearts and minds as well.

A protein-packed classic made lighter and better for you. Rich, creamy, and oh-so-satisfying!

This butter chicken was my weekend favorite growing up — creamy, spiced just right, and always made with love by my mom. I've recreated it with a nourishing twist, keeping the comfort while lightening it up. It's still a crowd-pleaser, now with ingredients that love you back.

the ultimate creamy butter chicken

Butter Chicken, also known as Chicken Tikka Masala or Chicken Butter Masala, is one of the most beloved Indian chicken dishes, renowned for its balanced flavors and rich, creamy sauce. It's a favorite in Indian restaurants and often one of the first dishes that comes to mind when you think of Indian cuisine.

ingredients

for the chicken marinade:
2 lbs boneless chicken thighs cut into bite-sized pieces
1 cup plain non-fat Greek yogurt
2 tbsp crushed fresh cilantro
1 tbsp lemon juice
2 tsp tandoori masala
1 tsp of fresh crushed ginger
1 tsp fresh crushed garlic
1 tsp red chili powder *(adjust to taste)*
1 tsp olive oil
1/2 tsp coriander powder
Salt according to taste

for the sauce:
1 cup chopped red onions *(approximately 2 medium onions)*
1 cup tomato puree
1 cup buttermilk
1 1/2 tbsp vegan butter
1 tbsp coriander powder
1/2 tbsp Kasthuri methi *(dried fenugreek leaves)*
1 tsp cumin seeds
1 tsp crushed fresh ginger
1 tsp crushed fresh garlic
1 tsp red chili powder *(adjust to taste)*
1 tsp garam masala
Salt according to taste

directions

Mix the marinade ingredients together in a large bowl and marinate the chicken for 6-8 hours, preferably overnight.

Take the marinated chicken out of the refrigerator 30 minutes prior to cooking to allow the yogurt to reach room temperature. Heat oil in a pan over medium heat and sauté the chicken until it is fully cooked and beautifully golden brown, which should take around 12-15 minutes. Remove the chicken and set it aside. In the same pan, melt butter and add cumin seeds, allowing them to splutter. Next, add the onions and sauté them over medium-high heat until they become soft and translucent. Then, incorporate the crushed ginger-garlic. Cook for a few more minutes. Add coriander powder, salt, red chili powder, and tomato puree to the pan. Stir well, cover with a lid, and let it simmer for another 12 minutes.

Add the cooked chicken and garam masala to the pan, stirring well, and let it simmer on low heat for 8 minutes. Next, pour in the buttermilk and cook for an additional 6-8 minutes. Once the sauce begins to simmer again, add kasthuri methi (dried fenugreek leaves) and let it cook for 7-9 minutes. Your butter chicken is now ready to serve! Enjoy it over fluffy basmati rice or warm naan for a complete meal.

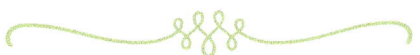

delicious butter chicken made right in your own kitchen!

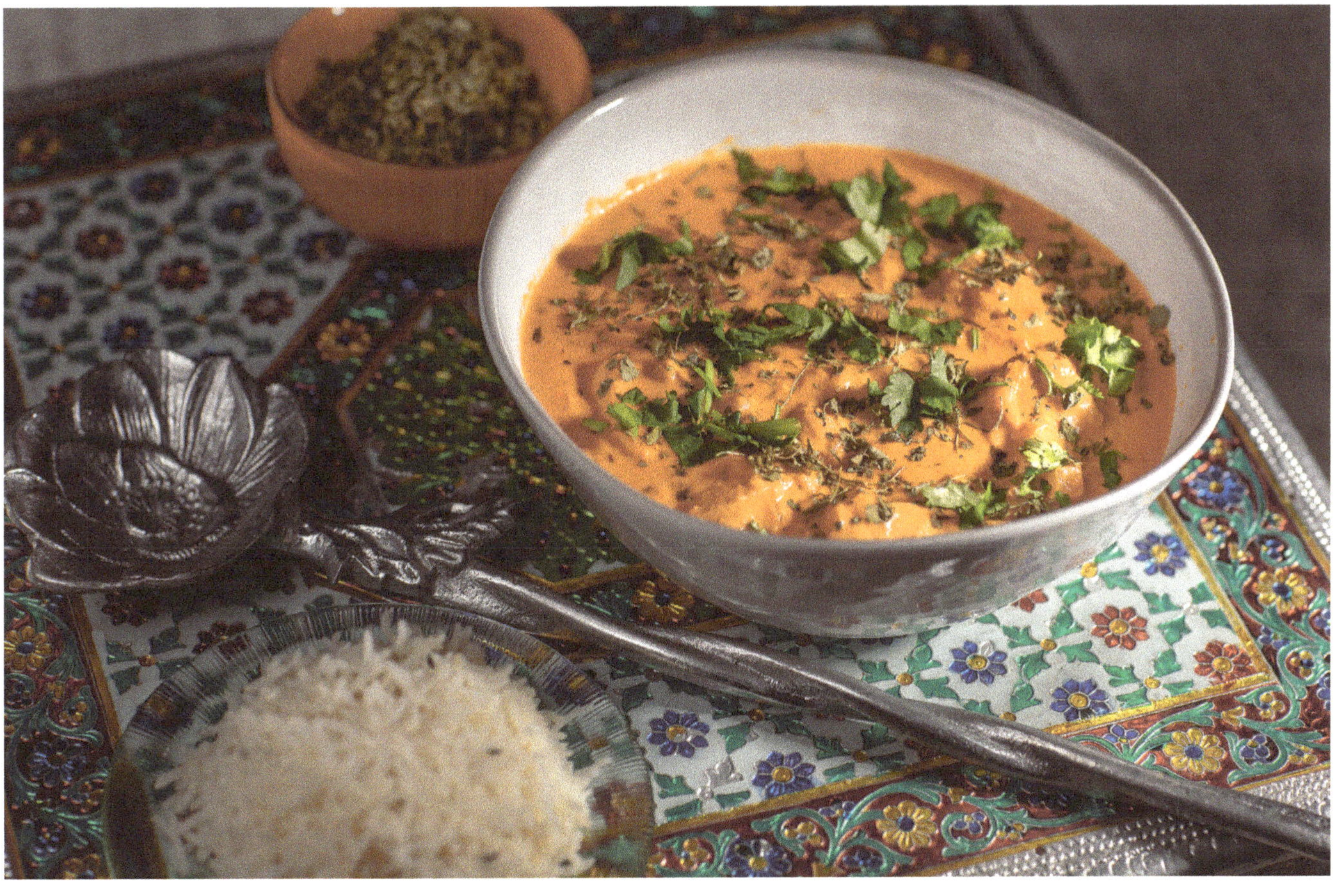

Rich, creamy, and bursting with flavor, you will enjoy preparing this classic Indian curry to serve at your table. It is perfectly paired with hot basmati rice or naan.

why I chose these ingredients

Better-for-you Butter Chicken: All the creamy, savory flavor—just made lighter, fresher, and perfect for your everyday table. Reimagined with a healthy twist! Enjoy the creamy goodness while nourishing your body with lean protein and immune-boosting spices!

buttermilk:
cool, calm, and cultured

Buttermilk is highly nutritious and offers numerous health benefits. It is an excellent source of minerals like calcium and potassium, as well as vitamins such as B12 and riboflavin. With lower fat and calorie content, it is a healthier option for those aiming to reduce fat intake. Its high protein content promotes satiety, aiding appetite control and weight management. Additionally, the probiotics in buttermilk support a healthy gut microbiome, which can strengthen the immune system.

greek yogurt:
your spoonful of strength

Greek yogurt is incredibly versatile, perfect for a range of dishes from smoothies and parfaits to savory sauces, making it a nutritious and easy addition to your diet. In butter chicken, Greek yogurt serves as an excellent marinade, adding extra protein and enhancing flavor. Packed with probiotics, it supports healthy digestion by promoting beneficial gut bacteria. With nearly twice the protein content of regular yogurt, Greek yogurt is ideal for muscle repair and growth while helping you stay full longer.

vegan butter:
a healthier, dairy-free choice

Vegan butter is a great alternative for people seeking a healthier option. Many vegan butters are lower in saturated fats compared to regular butter, which can be beneficial for heart health. Some use oils rich in unsaturated fats, such as olive, avocado, or coconut oil.

cumin seeds:
small seeds, big flavor

Cumin seeds are not only flavorful but also packed with numerous health benefits. India is one of the largest producers of cumin seeds in the world, particularly in regions like Gujarat and Rajasthan. Cumin's versatility as both a whole seed and ground spice makes it adaptable to a variety of cooking techniques, whether it's dry roasting for extra flavor, tempering for aroma, or using ground cumin in spice mixes. Cumin is beneficial for balancing digestion, detoxifying the body, and boosting immunity.

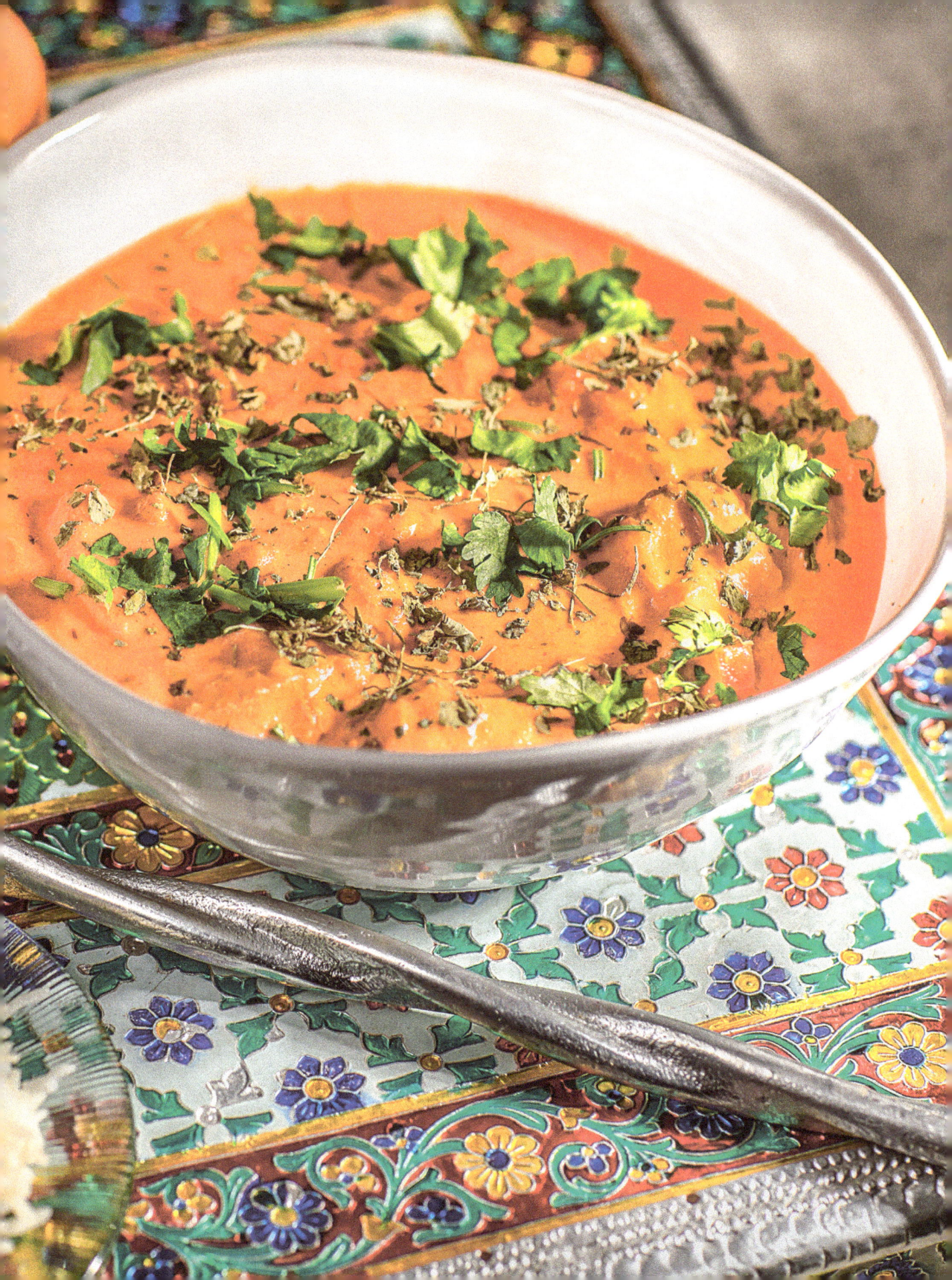

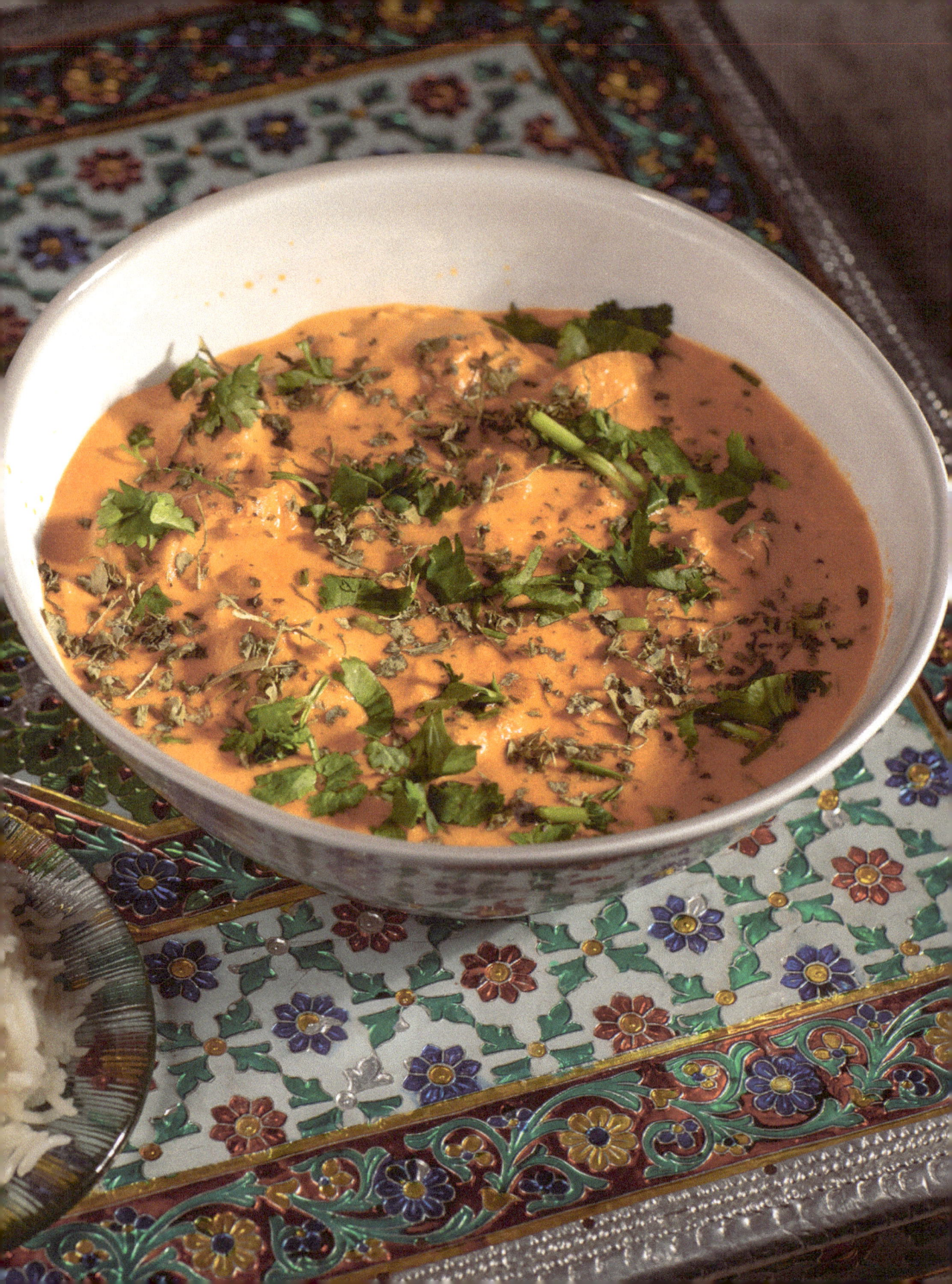

chicken tighs:
flavor meets nutrition

Chicken thighs bring rich flavor and juicy tenderness to this dish, thanks to their naturally higher fat content. This extra fat not only enhances taste but also keeps the meat moist without needing added oils—perfect for creating satisfying meals with minimal effort. The heartier profile of chicken thighs can help you feel fuller for longer, making them a great option for portion control and for those following a low-carb or higher-fat diet.

kasthuri methi:
a flavorful boost with health perks

Dried fenugreek leaves, also known as kasthuri methi, are a beloved staple in Indian cooking, often added to curries, stews, and savory dishes for their warm, nutty aroma and depth of flavor. I love using them to elevate the richness of a curry while adding a gentle earthiness. Beyond taste, they bring a lot to the table nutritionally, packed with vitamins A, C, and K, and minerals like iron, calcium, and magnesium. Their high fiber content helps promote a sense of fullness, aiding appetite control and supporting healthy weight management. Plus, their immune-supporting nutrients offer an extra reason to sprinkle them onto your meals

heat with heart:
red chili powder

I enjoy incorporating red chili powder into my recipes because of its health benefits. It is a good source of vitamins and minerals, including vitamin A, and vitamin B6, which are important for skin health, and energy metabolism. The high vitamin C content in red chili powder can enhance immune function, helping the body fight off infections. Besides turning up the flavor, this staple spice supports heart health and adds cultural flair to every bite

spice with purpose:
the magic of garam masala

Garam masala is a warm, aromatic blend of ground spices commonly used in Indian cuisine. It typically includes cinnamon, cloves, cardamom, cumin, coriander, black pepper, nutmeg, mace, and bay leaf. Each of these spices carries unique health benefits, but when combined, they create a powerful blend that is as nourishing as it is flavorful.
Adding garam masala to your meals can support digestion, as spices like cumin and coriander stimulate digestive enzymes and reduce bloating. The warming spices may also boost metabolism, helping your body process food more efficiently. Rich in antioxidants and anti-inflammatory compounds, this spice mix can help protect cells from damage and support overall immune health.
A small sprinkle goes a long way—not just in flavor, but in wellness too.

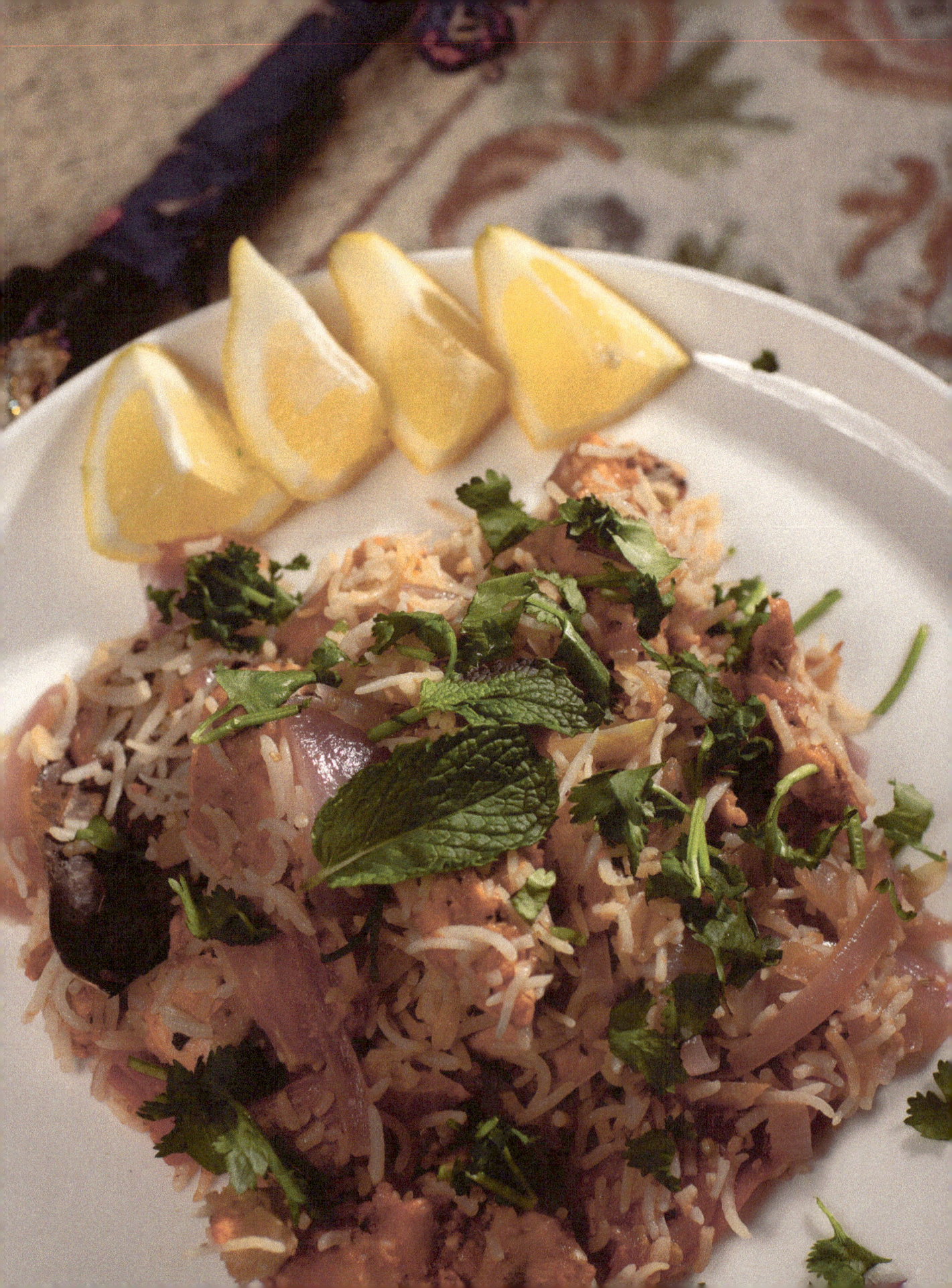

balanced chicken biryani feast

From fresh, wholesome ingredients to the careful process of bringing them together, each recipe is a celebration of the love, care, and joy that go into making a meal.

A fragrant one-pot wonder full of nourishing spices, protein & whole ingredients. Spiced to perfection, fueled with flavor!

This chicken biryani is more than just a meal—it's a family tradition wrapped in spice and love. It's comfort, connection, and love layered with spice.

balanced chicken biryani feast

Chicken biryani is a flavorful and aromatic dish originating from the Indian subcontinent. It is a beloved culinary classic with regional variations across India and beyond. It is a one-pot meal made by layering marinated chicken with basmati rice, spices, and herbs. A traditional biryani consists of fluffy basmati rice layered over tender and succulent pieces of any kind of meat, accompanied by the mesmerizing aromas of spices, herbs, and caramelized onions.

ingredients

for marination:
1 lb boneless chicken thighs
1/2 cup plain Greek yogurt
2 tbsp tandoori chicken masala
2 tbsp lemon juice
1 tbsp olive oil
1 tsp minced garlic
1 tsp crushed fresh ginger
1 tsp coriander powder
1/2 tsp cumin powder
1/2 tsp red chili powder
Salt according to taste

for making rice and onion tomato base:
1 cup basmati rice soaked for 3-4 hours
2 cups water
1 1/2 cup thinly sliced red onions
2 cups thinly sliced tomatoes
2 tbsp chopped cilantro
3 tsp olive oil
2 tsp ghee
3 pieces of bay leaves
1 tsp cumin seeds

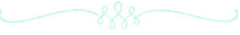

fluffy & fragrant

Soaking your rice beforehand helps it cook evenly and fluff up—keeping it light, airy, and easier to digest.

directions

Mix the marinade ingredients together in a large bowl and marinate the chicken for 6-8 hours, preferably overnight. Remove the chicken from the fridge before starting the biryani preparation. Bringing it closer to room temperature ensures even cooking and maintains its tenderness.

3 main steps to cooking chicken biryani:

Cooking the chicken: Heat 1 teaspoon of oil in a heavy bottomed pan, add the marinated chicken and cook until it turns golden brown on both sides. Cook the chicken in batches to ensure even cooking. Once done, set the chicken aside.

Cooking onion tomato base: Heat 2 teaspoons of ghee in the same pan, then toss in the garlic and ginger, cooking just until they release that delicious aroma. Add the onions and sauté until golden brown, then stir in the tomatoes and cook for 5–7 minutes. Season with a pinch of salt, then set the mixture aside—it is going to bring bold flavor to your next layer!

Cooking Rice: Take a pan or pot and heat 2 teaspoons of oil over medium heat. Add cumin seeds, bay leaves, and let them sizzle for about a minute until they release their

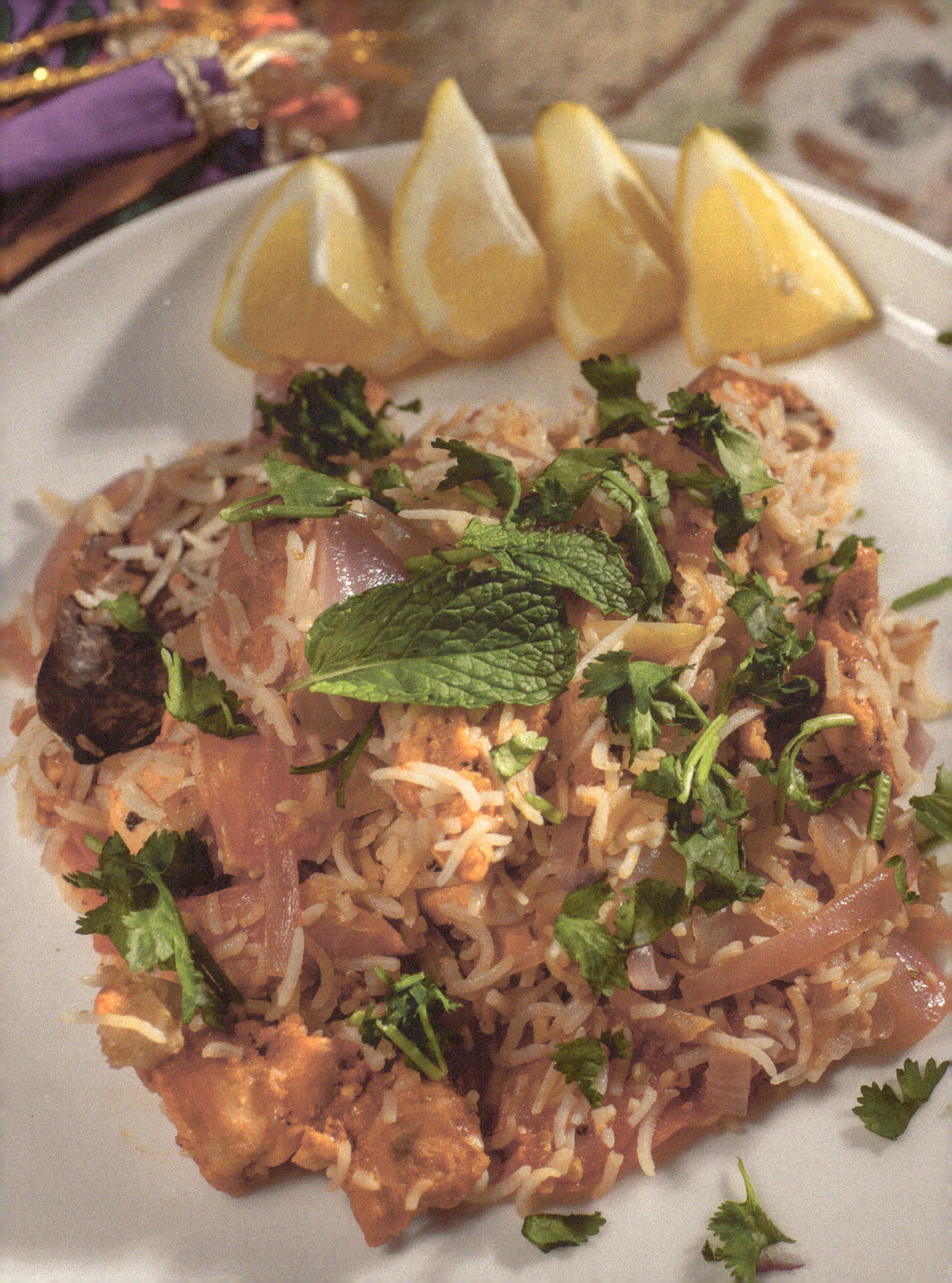

made to share

Packed with protein and tradition—
this dish brings both flavor and family to the table.

fragrance. Drain the soaked basmati rice and stir it into the pan. Cook on low heat for 5–10 minutes, stirring occasionally, until the grains are lightly golden and toasty.

Pour in the measured water and bring it to a gentle boil over high heat. Once boiling, reduce the heat to medium-low, cover, and cook until the water is absorbed, and the rice turns fluffy and fragrant.

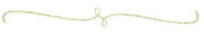

rice cooking tip

For fluffy and perfectly cooked basmati rice, use a 1:2 ratio—1 cup of rice to 2 cups of water. This balance allows the rice to absorb just the right amount of moisture, giving you soft, separate grains every time.

In the same pan you used for the onion-tomato base, start layering—begin with the rice, then the onion-tomato mixture, followed by the chicken. Repeat the layers until everything is in. Keep the heat on low and let it all simmer for 7–8 minutes to bring those flavors together. Sprinkle in the garam masala and cook for another 5–7 minutes. Finish with a fresh cilantro garnish... and just like that, your biryani is ready to serve.

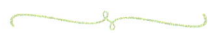

let's explore some benefits of adding ghee to your diet:

Ghee, a type of clarified butter commonly used in Indian and South Asian cuisines, is made by simmering butter to separate the milk solids and water from the fat. The result is a rich, golden-yellow liquid with a distinctive nutty flavor and aroma. Ghee is packed with fat-soluble vitamins such as A, D, E, and K, which are essential for immune health, bone strength, and other vital functions. It is also thought to promote digestion by stimulating the secretion of stomach acids. Despite concerns about saturated fats, moderate consumption of ghee may support heart health by improving cholesterol levels, particularly by raising HDL (good) cholesterol. Additionally, ghee is an excellent source of healthy fats, providing a steady source of energy.

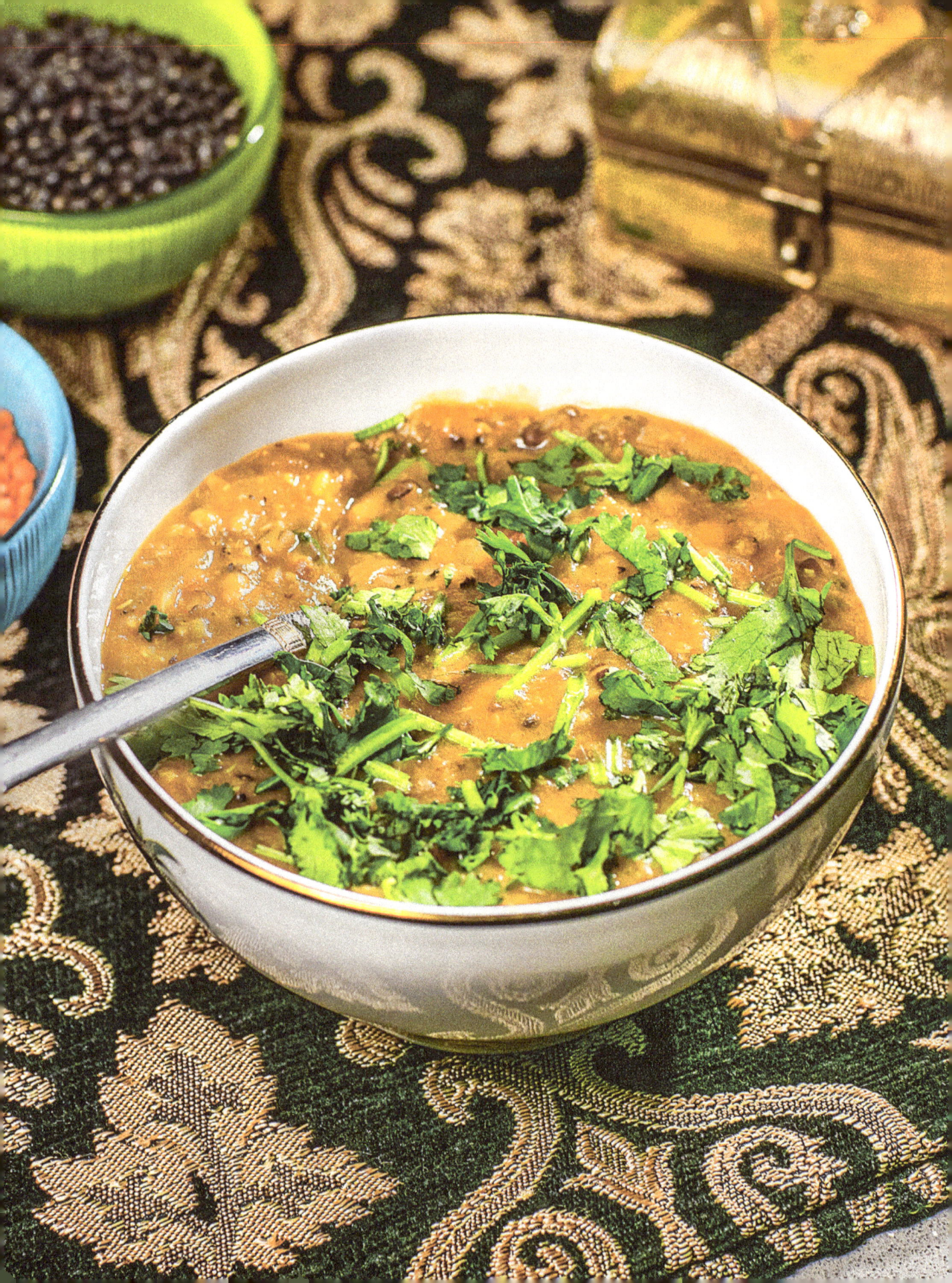

7-lentil harmony
curry soup

It's not just about cooking, it's about crafting something that fuels us, connects us, and reminds us of the beauty in simple, nutritious food.

Comfort in every spoonful. Today, as I prepare this lentil curry for my own family, I'm reminded of those moments—how food can be a bridge between generations, a way to pass down love, care, and tradition. This recipe, much like the ones I grew up with, has become a symbol of warmth, nourishment, and the beauty of simple, nutritious ingredients coming together in perfect harmony.

7-lentil harmony curry soup

Seven lentils, one extraordinary curry – packed with variety, flavor, and all the nutritional benefits your body craves! Why settle for one when you can enjoy the goodness of seven lentils in every bite?

ingredients

1 1/2 cups chopped tomatoes
1 cup chopped onion
4 tbsp toor dal *(lentil)*
4 tbsp yellow moong dal *(lentil)*
4 tbsp green moong dal *(lentil)*
4 tbsp chana dal *(lentil)*
3 tbsp black gram dal *(lentil)*
3 tbsp urad dal **(lentil)**
3 tbsp orange moong dal *(lentil)*
2 1/2 tbsp olive oil *(or ghee)*
1 tbsp chopped cilantro
1 tsp cumin seeds
1 tsp turmeric powder
1 tsp crushed fresh ginger
1 tsp minced garlic
1/2 tsp red chili powder
1/2 tsp coriander powder
1/2 tsp cumin powder
1/2 tsp garam masala
Salt according to taste

directions

You can cook lentils in several ways: using a pressure cooker, an Instant Pot, or a regular cooking pot on the stovetop.

preparing the dal for cooking:

Rinse the dal thoroughly under water to remove any dirt or impurities. Soak all the lentils for 7-8 hours, or preferably overnight, in 4 cups of water, then drain them. Once drained, place the lentils into your preferred cooking method and add 3 cups of water. (Note: This recipe uses 1 cup of dal. If you are making a larger batch, simply add 3 cups of water for each cup of dal.

Add salt, turmeric, and oil/ghee. The oil helps prevent the dal from foaming too much, and turmeric gives a nice color.

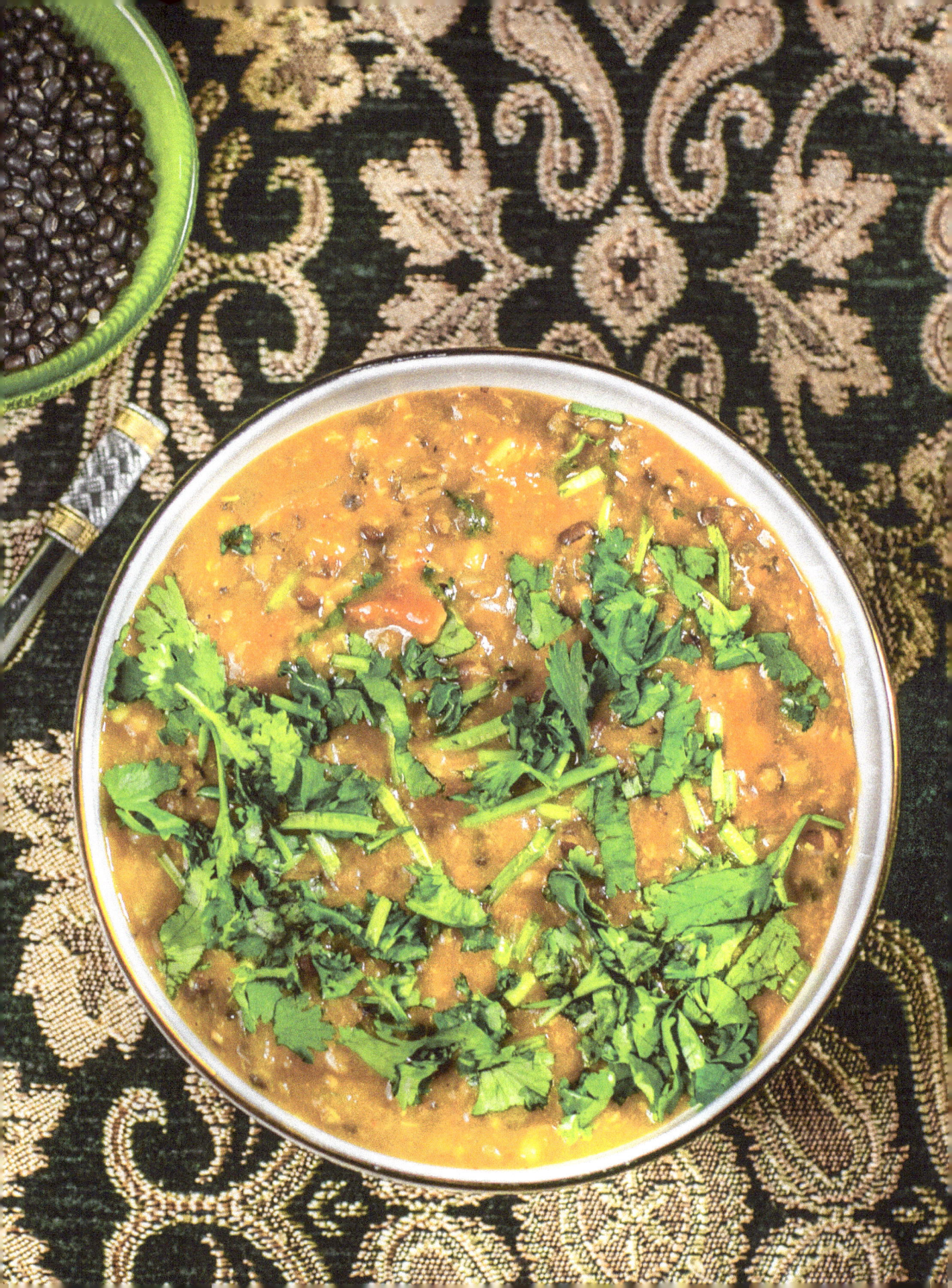

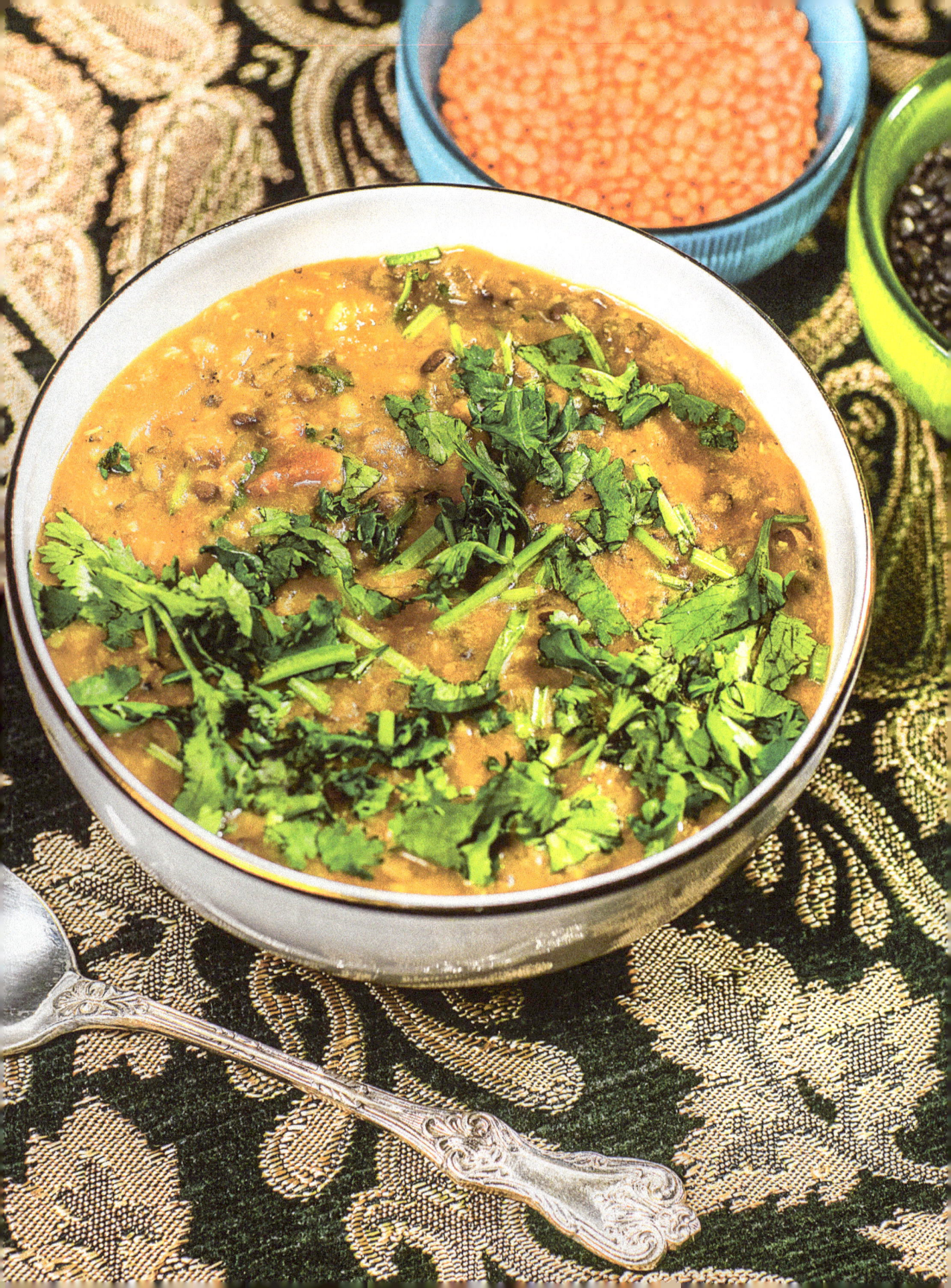

cooking the dal

pressure cooker

Add the lentils to the pressure cooker, secure the lid, and place the weight (whistle) on the vent. Cook on high heat until the first whistle, then reduce the heat to low and continue cooking for 3 more whistles. Turn off the heat and let the pressure release naturally for 5–7 minutes. Once the pressure is released, open the lid and stir the lentils well to mix everything evenly.

electric pressure cooker (instant pot)

If you are using an electric pressure cooker or Instant Pot, set it to cook on high pressure for 12–14 minutes. Once the timer goes off, let the pressure release naturally—no need to rush this part! When the lid unlocks, your lentils should be soft, and ready to stir.

regular pot

If you don't have a pressure cooker, you can easily cook lentils in a regular pot, just allow a bit of extra time, usually about 30 minutes. Make sure you still soaked the lentils. Bring water to a boil, then add the dal along with salt, turmeric, and a touch of oil or ghee. Once it is bubbling again, reduce the heat, partially cover the pot, and let it gently simmer for about 25–30 minutes. Stir occasionally, the dal should be tender and easy to mash with the back of a spoon.

preparing the lentil curry:

Heat oil in a frying pan over medium heat. Add cumin seeds and let them sizzle for a few seconds until fragrant. Stir in the garlic and ginger, Cook for a few seconds.

Add chopped onions and cook for 5-7 minutes until they turn transparent. Next, add the chopped tomatoes and cook for an additional 7-8 minutes.

Mix in red chili powder, coriander powder, turmeric powder, cumin powder, and salt. Stir everything together to form a flavorful masala base.

Add the cooked lentils to the mixture, cook on medium-high heat, and bring it to a boil. Sprinkle in garam masala, reduce the heat, and let it simmer for 10–15 minutes. If the dal thickens too much, add a splash of water to keep it creamy without making it too runny.

Finish by garnishing with fresh cilantro and serve hot with fluffy white rice or warm roti!

one pot, seven pulses, infinite comfort

India has a long-standing tradition of incorporating lentils into its cuisine, where they are not only a rich source of protein but also hold cultural and nutritional significance. Whether skinned, split, or pureed, lentils have been a beloved ingredient in Indian dishes for centuries, dating back to 2500 B.C.

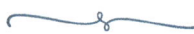

I love lentils and decided to experiment by mixing different varieties to explore how their flavors and textures would come together. It turned out to be one of my best culinary ideas, it was absolutely delicious! The combination of seven types of lentils, each offering unique nutrients, paired with a medley of spices, onions, and tomatoes, created a rich, flavorful experience in every bite. It quickly became one of my favorite meals to make and share!

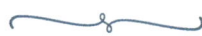

In Hindi, lentils are called 'dal,' and they are a staple in many Indian kitchens. The word 'dal' refers not just to the lentil itself but also to the dishes made from these nutritious legumes. In this recipe, we are using a variety of lentils (or dal) to create a hearty, flavorful curry that is rich in protein and full of traditional Indian spices.

Lentil curry soup is considered healthy for several reasons:

rich in nutrients

Packed with Goodness, lentils are little powerhouses loaded with plant-based protein, fiber, folate, iron, and magnesium—fueling your body with the nutrients it needs to thrive

high in protein

Lentils are an excellent plant-based protein source, making them a great option for vegetarians and vegans. They provide the protein necessary for muscle repair and growth.

fiber-fueled health

Lentils are high in fiber, which promotes healthy digestion, supports weight management, and helps regulate blood sugar by slowing down the absorption of carbohydrates.

support heart health

Lentils are naturally low in fat, making lentil curry a heart-healthy choice. Their rich content of fiber, potassium, and antioxidants supports heart health by helping to reduce blood pressure and maintain healthy cholesterol levels.

anti-inflammatory properties

Many spices used in lentil curry, such as turmeric and ginger, have anti-inflammatory properties, which can help reduce inflammation in the body

hydration

As a soup, lentil curry is hydrating, which is important for overall health, especially in maintaining proper digestion and skin health.

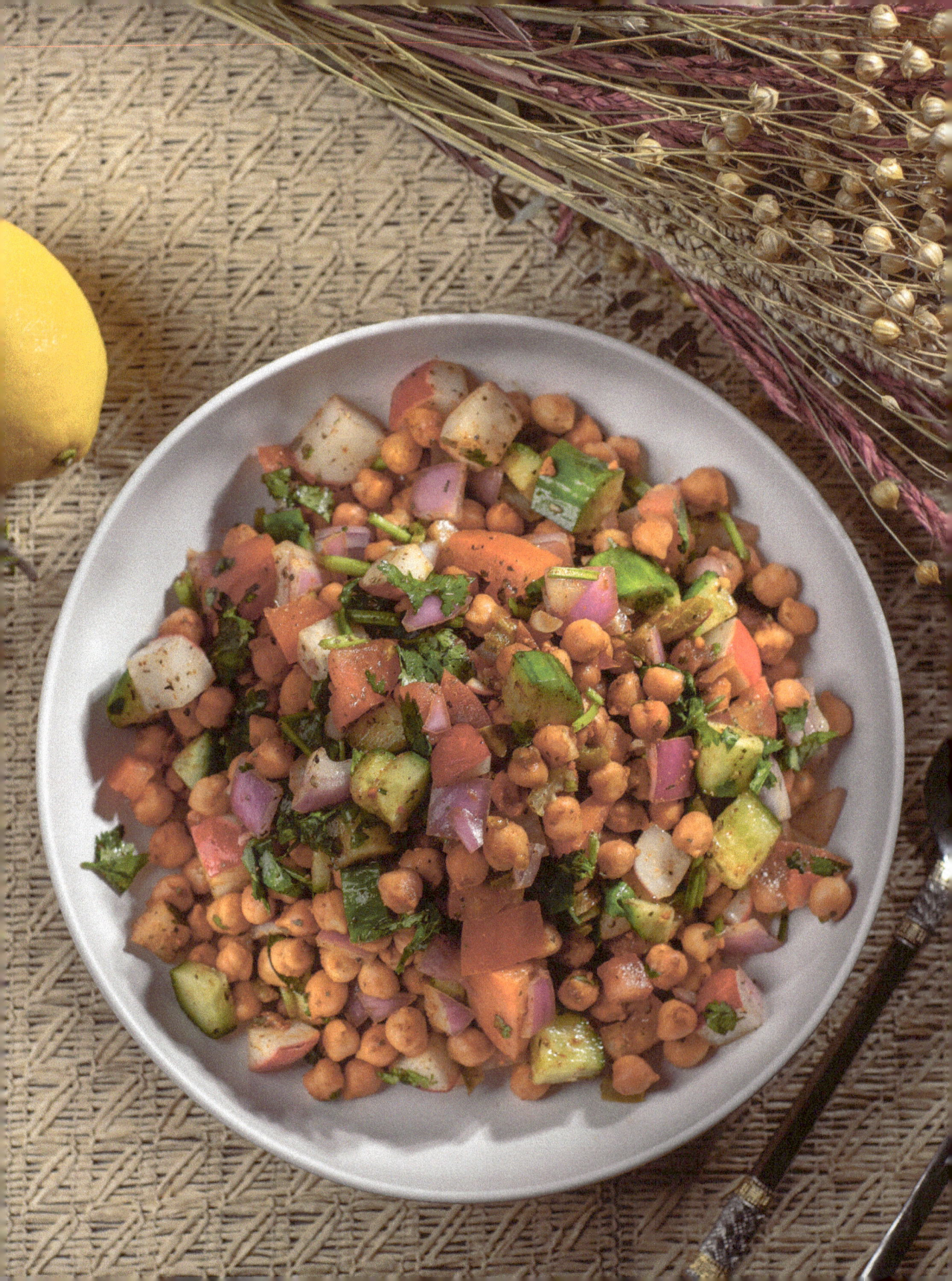

chickpea curry salad

In the kitchen, the magic happens when you take the time to select ingredients that are vibrant, fresh, and full of life. Each vegetable, each herb, and every grain has its own story to tell, and when combined, they create something far greater than the sum of their parts.

Zingy, satisfying, and full of flavor. A vibrant bowl of fiber, protein, and spice that satisfies every craving. This fresh salad is a perfect example of how salads can be both nourishing and delicious. When the mood calls for something hearty yet nutritious, the Chickpea Curry Salad is always my first choice—a powerhouse of nutrition with a delightful crunch.

chickpea curry salad

This recipe came to life late one night in my kitchen when I was starving. I raided the fridge, grabbed some healthy ingredients, and thought, why not mix these together and see what happens? The result was one of the tastiest creations I have ever made!

ingredients

2 1/2 cups garbanzo beans *(aka chickpeas)*
1/2 cup chopped red onions
1/2 cup chopped cucumber
1/2 cup chopped red radish
1/2 cup chopped tomatoes *(any kind)*
1/4 cup chopped mint leaves
1/4 cup chopped cilantro
4-5 tbsp red wine vinegar
1 tbsp olive oil
1/2 tbsp chopped fresh garlic
1/2 tsp chopped jalapeno peppers *(pickled)*
1/4 tsp dried dill
1/4 tsp tandoori masala
(found in Indian grocery stores)
1/4 tsp coriander powder
Salt and pepper according to taste

directions

Heat olive oil in a large skillet over medium heat. Add the chopped garlic and sauté for about 30 seconds, just until fragrant.

Add the garbanzo beans into the skillet and cook for 4-5 minutes, allowing them to get slightly golden.

Add tandoori masala and coriander powder, give it a good stir, then cover and let it simmer on low heat for another 5–6 minutes.

As the spices blend in, the beans will take on a rich orange hue. Once done, turn off the heat and let the mixture cool slightly.

In a large mixing bowl, combine sauteed chickpeas and all the remaining ingredients, including the herbs and red wine vinegar. Stir everything together until it is well coated and vibrant.

Pop the bowl in the fridge for 10–15 minutes to let all those flavors mingle and settle in. Then dig in and enjoy!

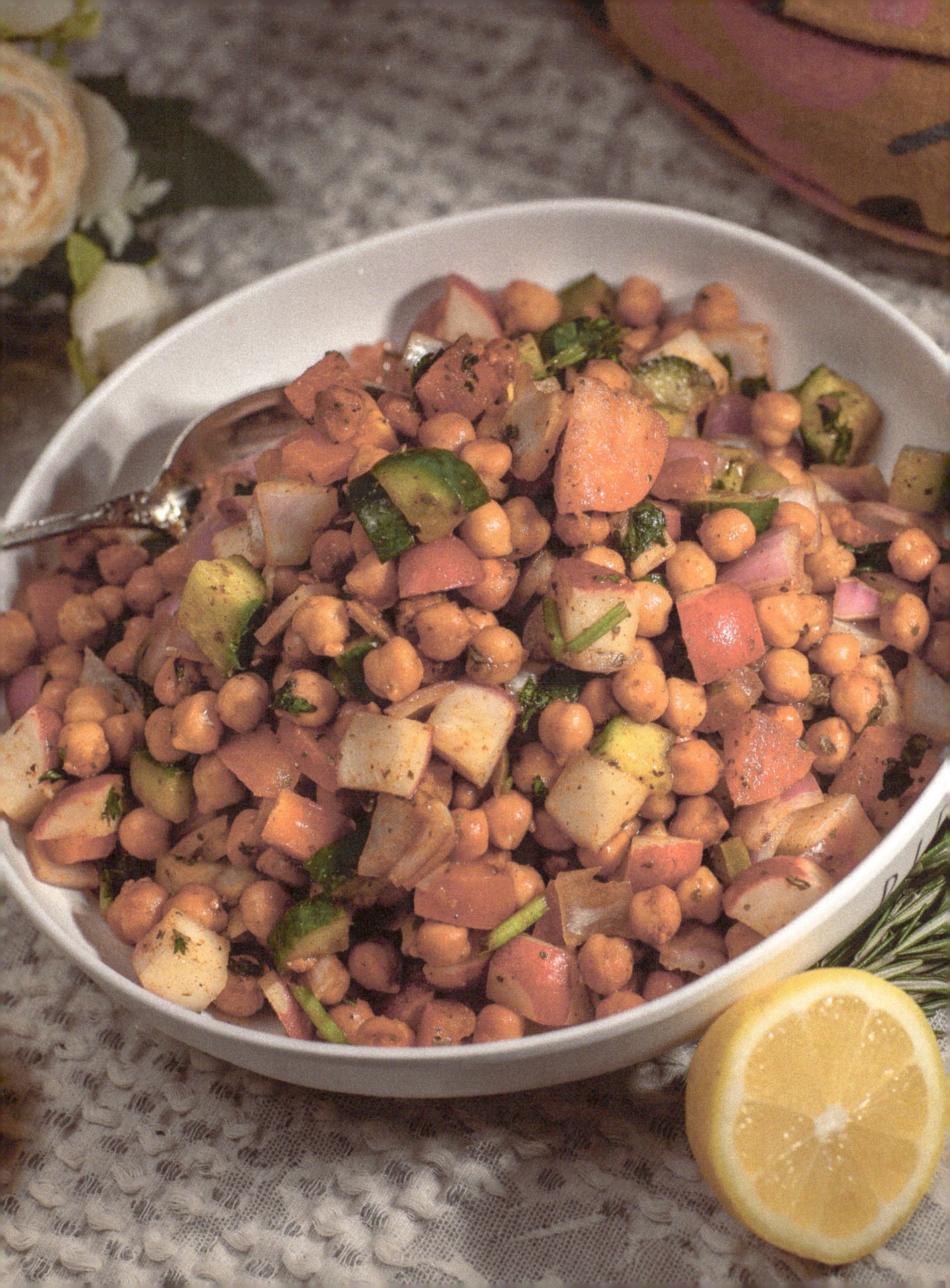

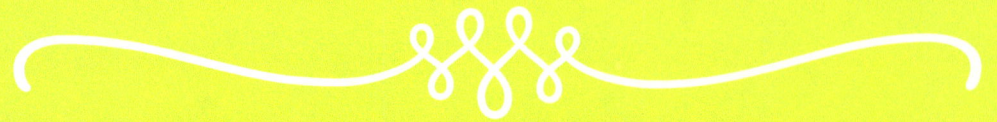

I love how the spices and fresh ingredients complement each other perfectly. The freshness and crispness really set this salad apart, making it truly one of a kind.

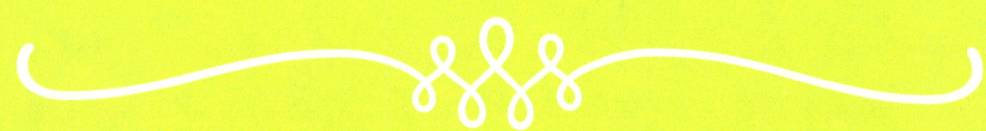

chickpea charm:

This recipe is both refreshing and ideal for enjoying as leftovers. Let me take a moment to explain why I have chosen each ingredient and how they play a vital role in our diet. These wholesome, natural foods are all about supporting a healthy lifestyle and offering long-term benefits for our bodies.

chickpea

Chickpeas are little powerhouses of plant-based protein and fiber, packed with iron, magnesium, and folate. Their mild, nutty flavor makes them the perfect canvas for spices, which is exactly why they have earned a spot in this dish!

red radish

Radishes are not just crunchy and colorful, they are gut-friendly too! Packed with fiber, they help keep digestion smooth and regular. Plus, their high-water content and anti-inflammatory compounds like anthocyanins offer a refreshing boost for your body from the inside out.

cilantro

Cilantro, also known as coriander leaves, is packed with health benefits. It is an excellent source of vitamins A, C, and K, as well as folate, potassium, and manganese, making it a nutrient-dense addition to any dish.

mint

Mint does more than freshen things up! It is rich in vitamins A and C, plus minerals like calcium, iron, and magnesium. Known for its calming touch, mint can ease digestion and help with bloating and discomfort—making it as healing as it is refreshing.

a salad that does it all

red onions

Red onions bring the crunch and the nutrients! Packed with antioxidants, they support heart health, digestion, fight inflammation and may even help balance blood sugar levels. A simple way to add both zing and nutrition to your meals!

cucumber

Cucumbers are a hydrating and nutritious vegetable, low in calories and high in vitamins K, C, and B. They support weight loss and promote healthy skin.

dill

Dill isn't just a flavorful herb—it is packed with nutrients too! Loaded with calcium and vitamin K for strong bones, and vitamin C to boost immunity, dill also supports digestion and adds a fresh twist to your favorite dishes.

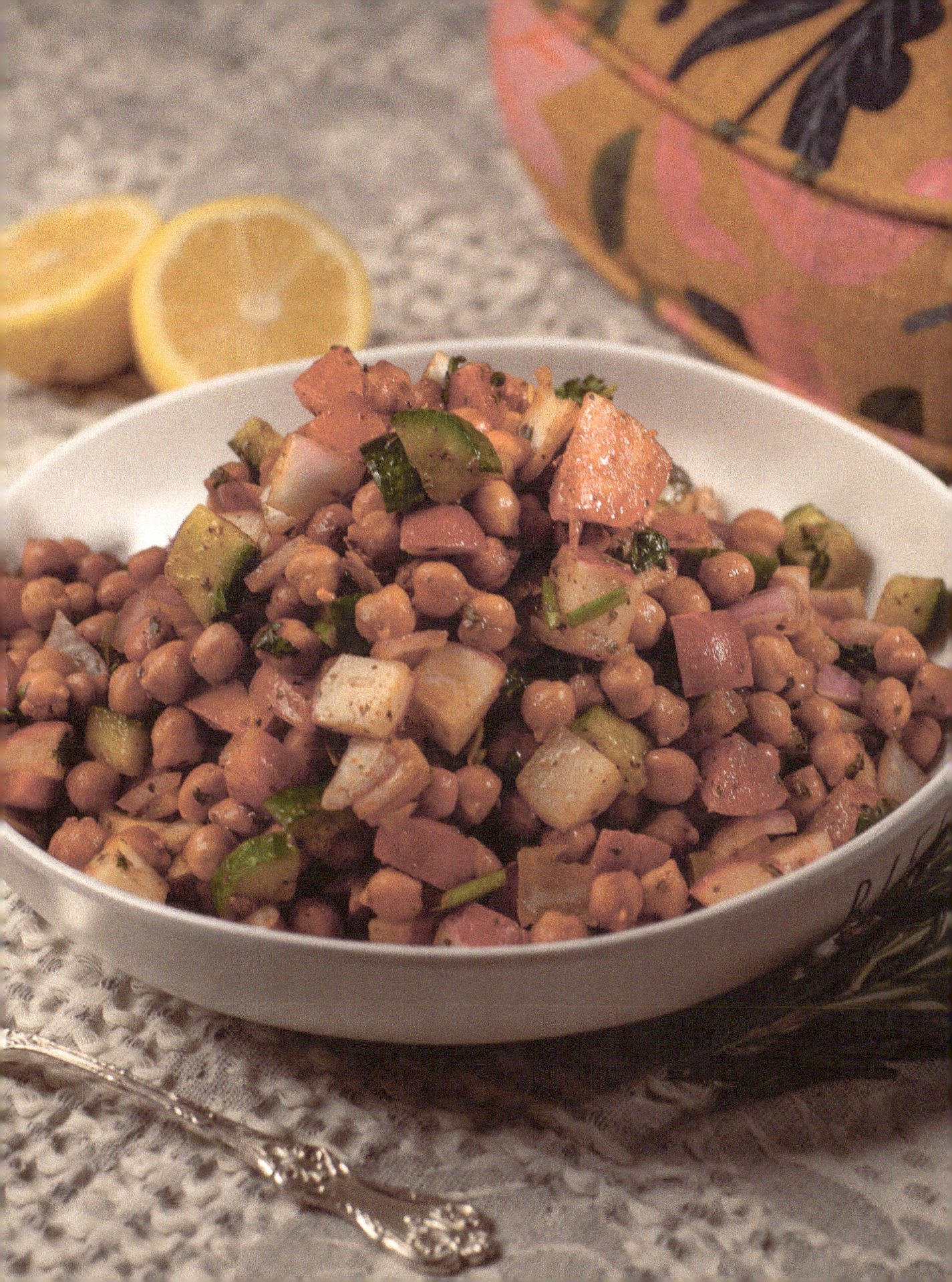

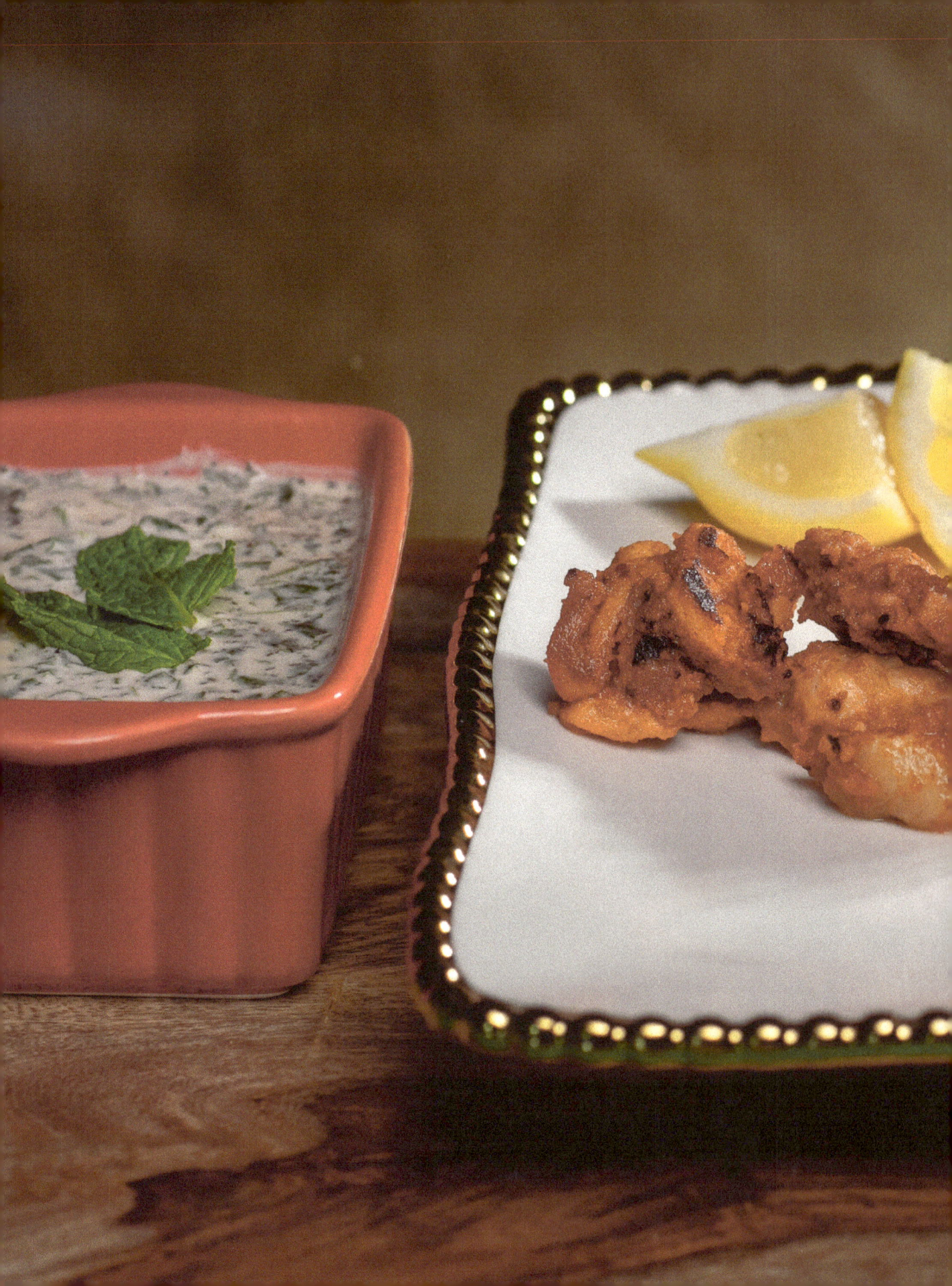

malai chicken kebab
with herb-infused white sauce

Each ingredient is a gift from the earth, and every step in the cooking process becomes an opportunity to honor the seasons and the cycles of life. As I chop, stir, and simmer, I'm reminded of the farmers, the soil, and the sun that helped bring these ingredients to life. In a world that often feels rushed, cooking gives us a chance to slow down, connect with what's real and nourishing, and appreciate the simple beauty of fresh, wholesome food.

Tender, creamy, and grilled to perfection. Cooked with probiotic-rich yogurt and aromatic spices. These kebabs are a beautiful blend of creamy yogurt marination and bold spices, and they always remind me of weekend cookouts with friends and family, gathering around to enjoy food and laughter.

malai chicken kebab with herb-infused white sauce

You are going to love these chicken kebabs! I have always been a fan of the magic that Greek yogurt and Indian spices bring together, and when you combine them to marinate juicy chicken, it's pure perfection. The result? Tender, flavorful kebabs with a creamy, spiced kick that you won't be able to stop at just one. Trust me, this recipe has become one of my go-to favorites, and once you taste them, you will wonder why you didn't try this sooner.

ingredients

for malai chicken kebab:
1 lb chicken thighs, boneless, cut into small pieces
1/2 cup plain Greek yogurt
1/4 cup buttermilk
4 tbsp chopped cilantro
3 tbsp white vinegar
2 tbsp olive oil
1 1/2 tbsp crushed garlic
2 tsp vegan butter
2 tsp garam masala powder
1 tsp crushed ginger
1 tsp coriander powder
1 tsp cumin powder
1 tsp chaat masala
Salt according to taste
2 lemons or limes cut into small pieces

directions

To make this flavorful kebab recipe, start by washing and cleaning your boneless chicken pieces. Pat them dry with a paper towel—this helps the marinade stick better. In a mixing bowl, combine salt, vinegar, ginger, garlic, Greek yogurt, cumin powder, coriander powder, and the rest of your marinade ingredients. Stir well until everything is blended smoothly.

Add the chicken to the bowl and mix until each piece is thoroughly coated. Cover and refrigerate overnight to let those rich flavors soak in.

The next morning, take the bowl out of the fridge and gently press each chicken piece between your palms to remove any excess marinade—this helps with even cooking. Set the pieces aside while you prepare your oven or grill.

Cut butter into small chunks and place it in a microwave-safe bowl to melt evenly.

Preheat the oven to 450°F (or alternately you can cook them on a barbeque grill). If you are using wooden skewers, soak them in water for about 30 minutes to prevent burning while cooking. Take a skewer and thread a chicken piece through it, ensuring it goes through the center to keep the chicken secure. Lightly spray a baking tray with olive oil and arrange the skewers on it, bake for 12-15 minutes. Remove the tray, brush the kebabs with melted butter, flip them over, and bake for another 10 minutes until they are golden, juicy, and cooked through.

Once done, carefully remove the skewers and place them on a serving plate. Garnish with a sprinkle of chaat masala and a squeeze of lemon juice.

The Malai Chicken Kebab is ready!

> Whether you are cooking for a special occasion or just treating yourself, these kebabs will be the star of your meal.

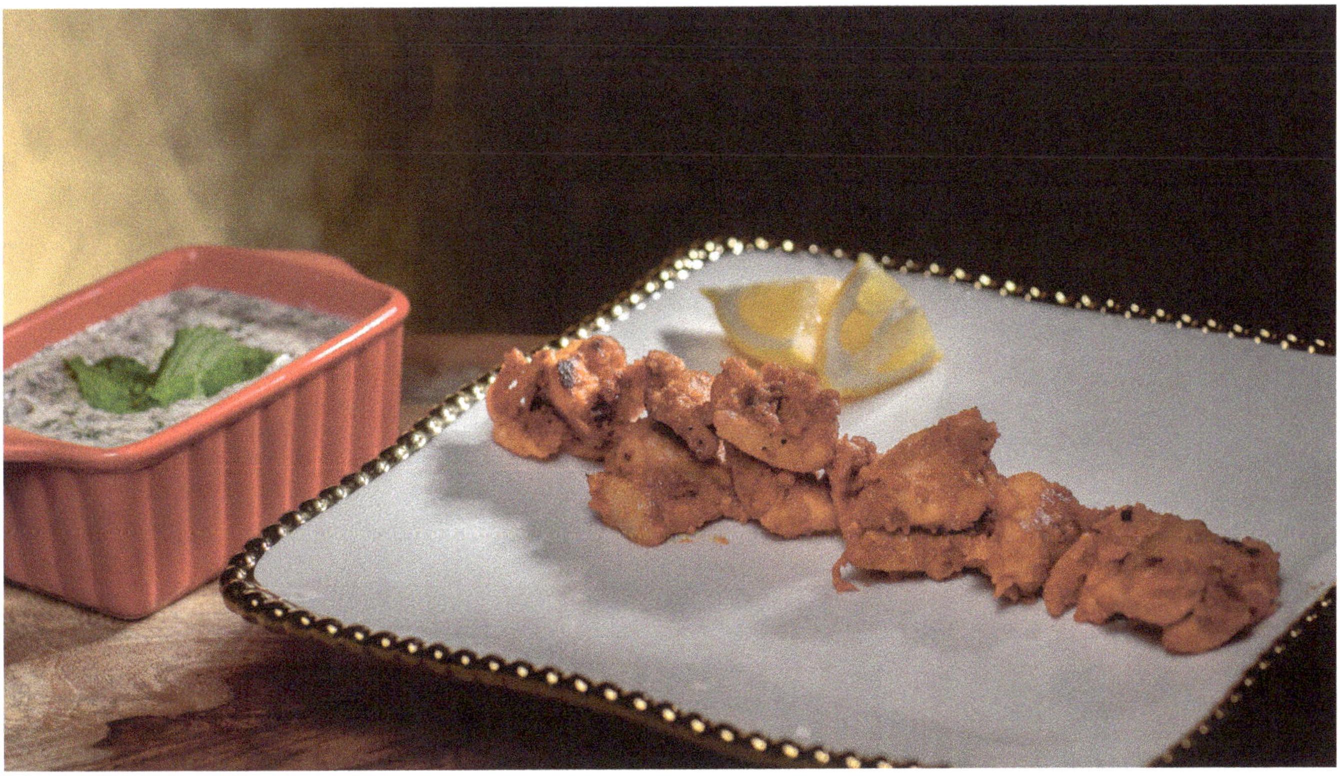

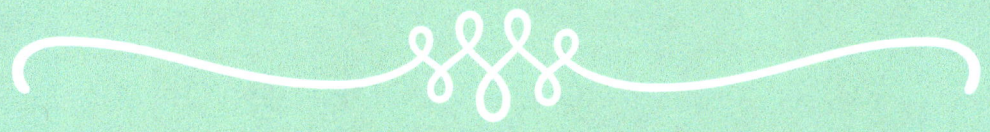

low-carb, high flavor

Perfect for those watching their carbs, these kebabs are a flavorful, low-carb option that won't sacrifice taste.

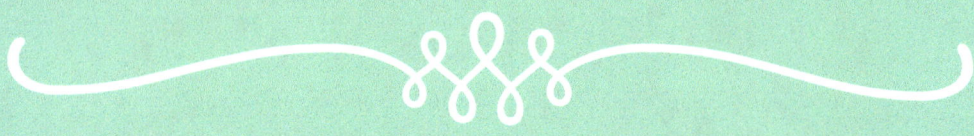

ingredients

for herb-infused white sauce:
1 cup Greek yogurt
3 tbsp fresh cilantro
3 tbsp fresh mint
1 tbsp extra virgin olive oil
3 tsp red wine vinegar
1/2 tsp dried dill
1/2 tsp crushed garlic
1/2 tsp black pepper
1/2 tsp siracha sauce (or more as desired)
1/2 tsp roasted cumin powder
1/2 tsp coriander powder
Salt according to taste

directions

In a bowl, combine the yogurt, cumin powder, coriander powder, and red wine vinegar. Add crushed garlic, sriracha sauce, olive oil, salt, black pepper, dried dill, and fresh herbs. Stir until everything is well combined. Cover and refrigerate overnight to let the flavors deepen and the herbs infuse their aroma.

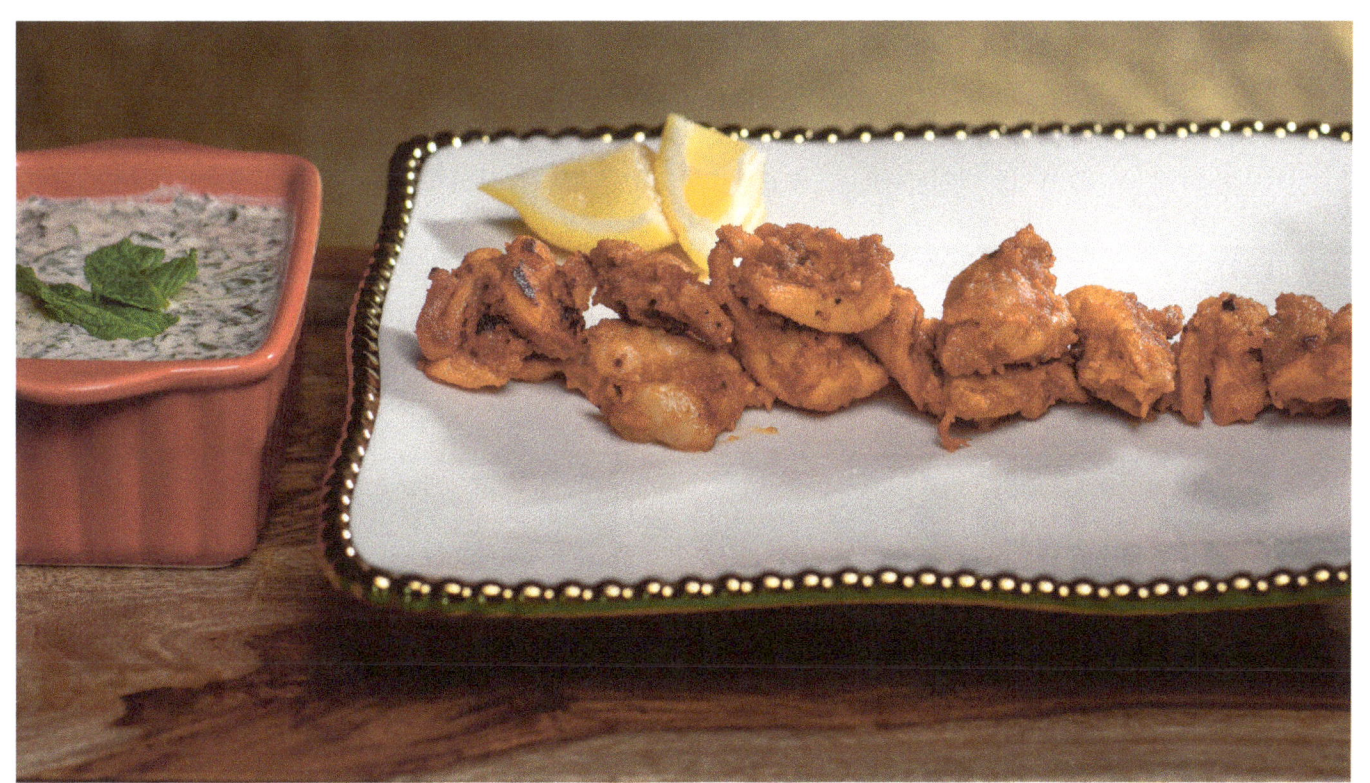

Greek yogurt and Indian spices— where flavor meets health!

Marinated in Greek yogurt and a mix of vibrant Indian spices, this recipe not only packs incredible flavor but also offers a great boost of protein, probiotics, and essential vitamins. Greek yogurt provides gut-friendly probiotics and calcium, while the spices like turmeric and cumin add anti-inflammatory benefits. It is a deliciously wholesome dish that is perfect for anyone looking to enjoy a meal that's both nutritious and bursting with flavor. I can't wait for you to try it and experience how the flavors and health benefits come together.

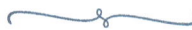

To elevate this dish, I pair it with a refreshing herb-infused white sauce that not only adds a zesty, fresh twist but also brings along a wealth of health benefits. Packed with antioxidants and anti-inflammatory properties from herbs like mint, cilantro, and dill, this sauce is as nourishing as it is delicious! It's the perfect balance of indulgence and wellness.

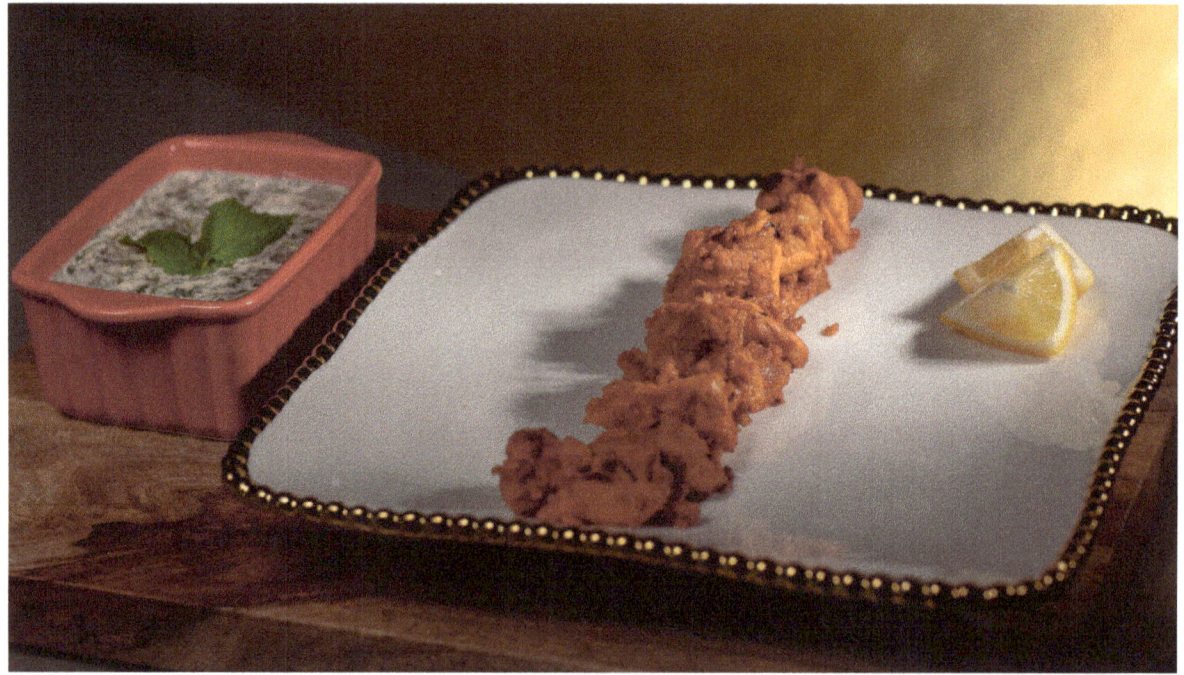

instant street food vibes—
chaat masala

Chaat masala is that zesty Indian spice blend that gives street food its irresistible kick! Made with bold ingredients like black salt, amchur (dried mango powder), cumin, coriander, and a touch of chili, it brings tang, salt, and spice to savory dishes.

> Black Salt is known in Ayurveda to improve digestion and balance electrolytes.

A spice that is great for your gut health! Packed with traditional ingredients like cumin and amchur, chaat masala doesn't just taste amazing, it supports digestion too. Chaat masala brings a nostalgic street-food vibe plus natural gut-loving ingredients like black salt and dried mango.

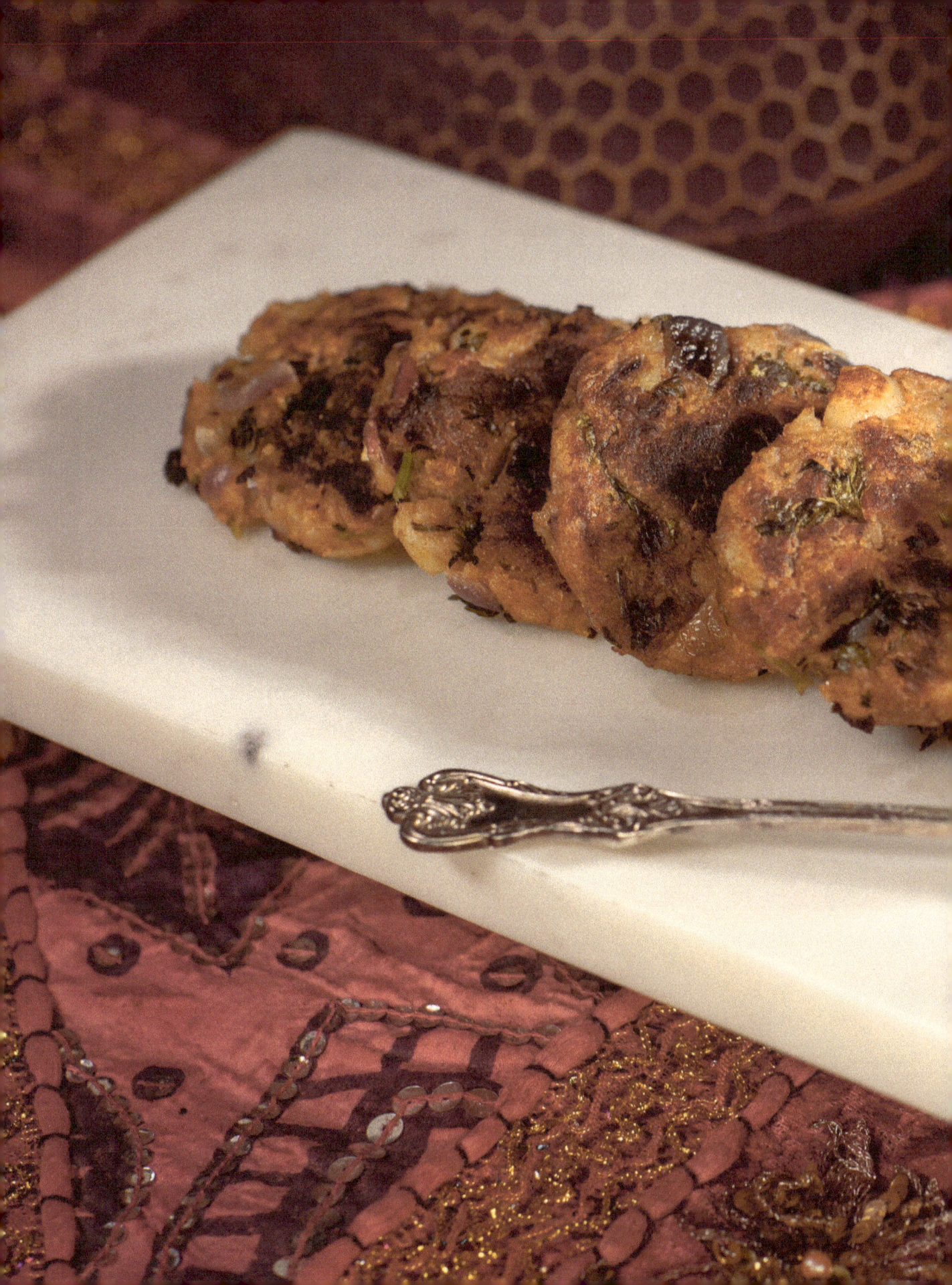

crispy aloo tikki
with mint chutney

It's in these simple, everyday rituals that we find something deeper—comfort, care, and a sense of home. Each recipe in this book carries with it the warmth of tradition and the excitement of nourishing our bodies with intention.

Fiber-rich, spiced to perfection, and totally snackable. Crispy on the outside, soft on the inside—these Aloo Tikkis take me straight back to childhood afternoons filled with street food cravings and laughter. Each bite is a warm, spiced hug that brings comfort and joy.

crispy aloo tikki with mint chutney

Aloo tikki, or potato cakes, are made with onions, chilies, herbs, and spices. It is one of those traditional snacks that never fails to impress me. They are simple yet incredibly clever in their flavor profile. Cooling fresh herbs balance the bold, pungent spices, while onions and green chilies add texture to the mashed potatoes. My recipe takes it a step further by introducing an optional crispy breadcrumb coating for added contrast.

ingredients

3 1/2 cups boiled mashed red potatoes *(approximately 5-6 medium sized potatoes)*
1/2 cup breadcrumbs *(whole wheat)*
1/2 cup chopped red onions
1/2 cup finely chopped cilantro
3 tbsp olive oil *(or oil spray)*
2 tsp finely chopped green chilies *(optional)*
1 tsp amchur powder *(dry mango powder)*
1 1/2 tsp red chili powder
1 1/2 tsp grated fresh ginger
1 tsp cumin powder
Salt and pepper according to taste

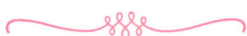

Aloo tikki is a perfect combination of crispy and soft textures, and when paired with refreshing mint chutney, it becomes a delightful snack. The mint chutney not only enhances the flavors but also provides a cool, tangy contrast to the warmth of the spiced potato cakes.

P.S: Mint chutney recipe on page 57.

directions

Wash and boil the potatoes, then mash them while they're still warm with the skin on for extra fiber and flavor. Add in your spices and knead the mixture thoroughly. Taste and adjust salt or seasonings as needed, then mix in the breadcrumbs until everything is well combined.

Cover the mixture and refrigerate it for 30-35 minutes.

Take a portion of the mixture in your hand, roll it into a ball, and then flatten it into a patty shape. (If the mixture is sticky, lightly oil your hands to shape it).

Heat oil in a pan over medium heat. Shallow fry the patties until they're golden brown and crisp on the outside. (Ensure the oil is at the right temperature—if it's too cold, the patties will absorb oil; if too hot, the outside will cook too quickly).

Place the aloo tikki on a paper towel to drain excess oil. Serve alongside mint chutney.

This recipe yields approximately 8-10 potato cakes, with a typical serving size of 2 per person. To serve more than 5 people, you can simply double the ingredient quantities.

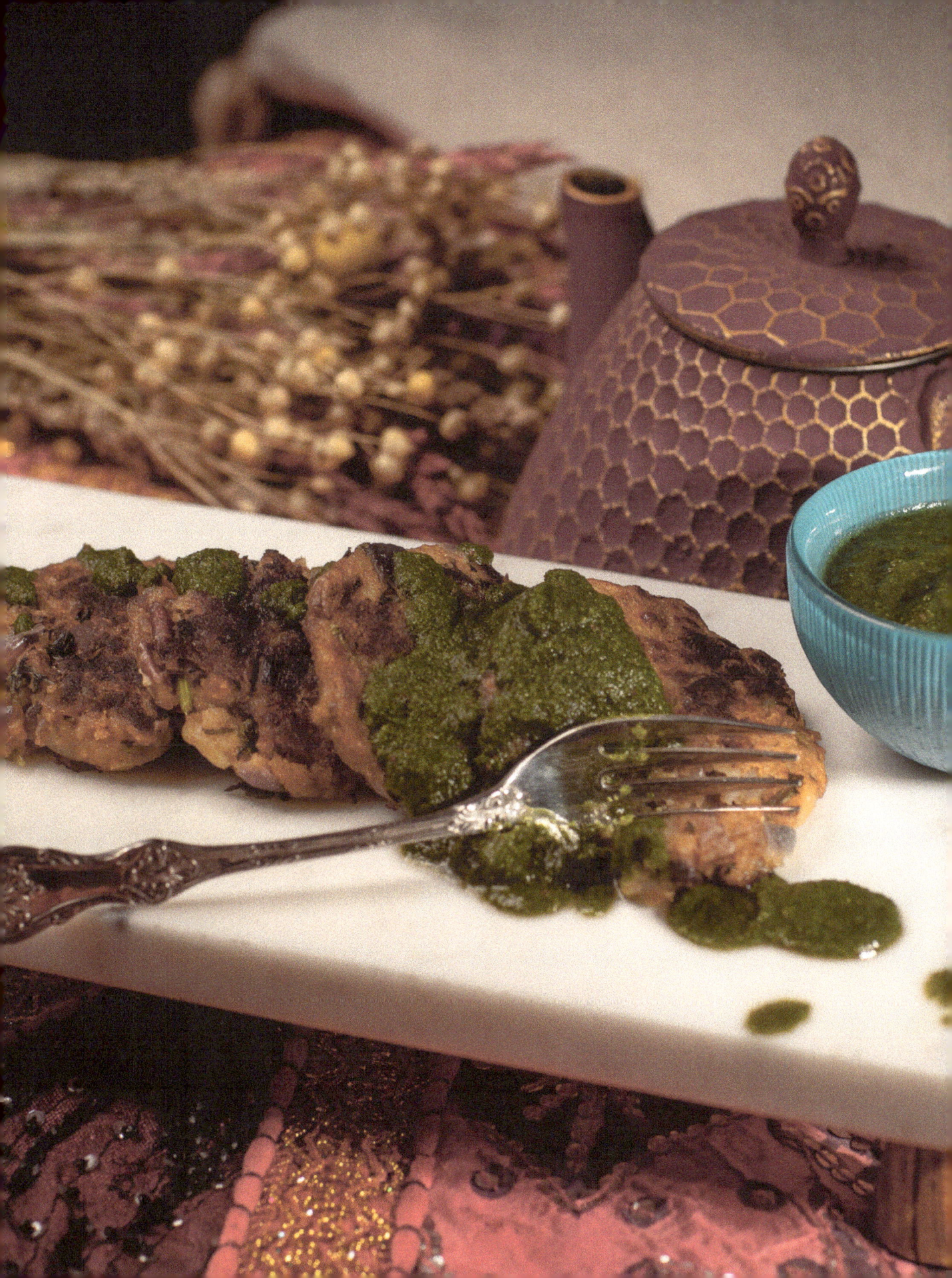

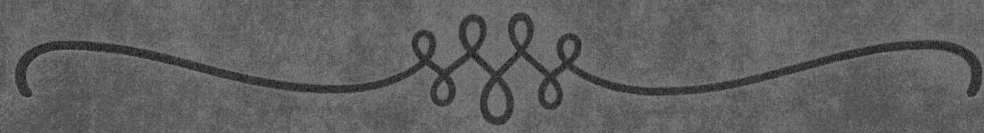

naturally vegan

A perfect choice for plant-based eaters. Keeping the skin on your potatoes adds extra fiber and nutrients, making your dish even more wholesome! Plus, it adds a nice texture and earthy flavor that complements the spices beautifully.

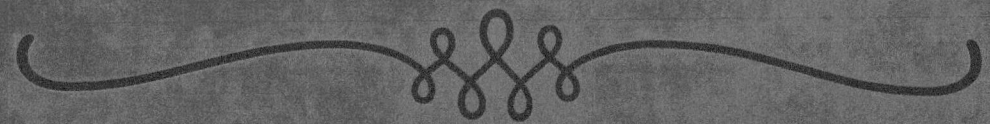

ingredient spotlight:
amchoor (dry mango powder)

If you spotted dry mango powder in the ingredient list and thought, "What's that?", you're not alone! Amchoor is one of my go-to secret spices. Made from dried green mangoes, it adds a tangy, citrusy kick that wakes up the flavors in a dish—without adding any extra moisture.

I love using it when I want that subtle sour note, especially in dals, chickpeas, or veggie stir-fries. It's not just about flavor either—amchoor is rich in antioxidants and vitamin C, and it's been used for ages in Ayurvedic cooking to aid digestion.

Here's why it's so loved in Indian cooking—and why it deserves a spot in your spice drawer:

flavor booster

A little goes a long way. It instantly brightens up dishes with a sour note, similar to lemon or tamarind, but dry and mellow.

versatile uses

Sprinkle on roasted veggies, toss into lentils or curries, or mix into spice blends like chaat masala for an extra zing.

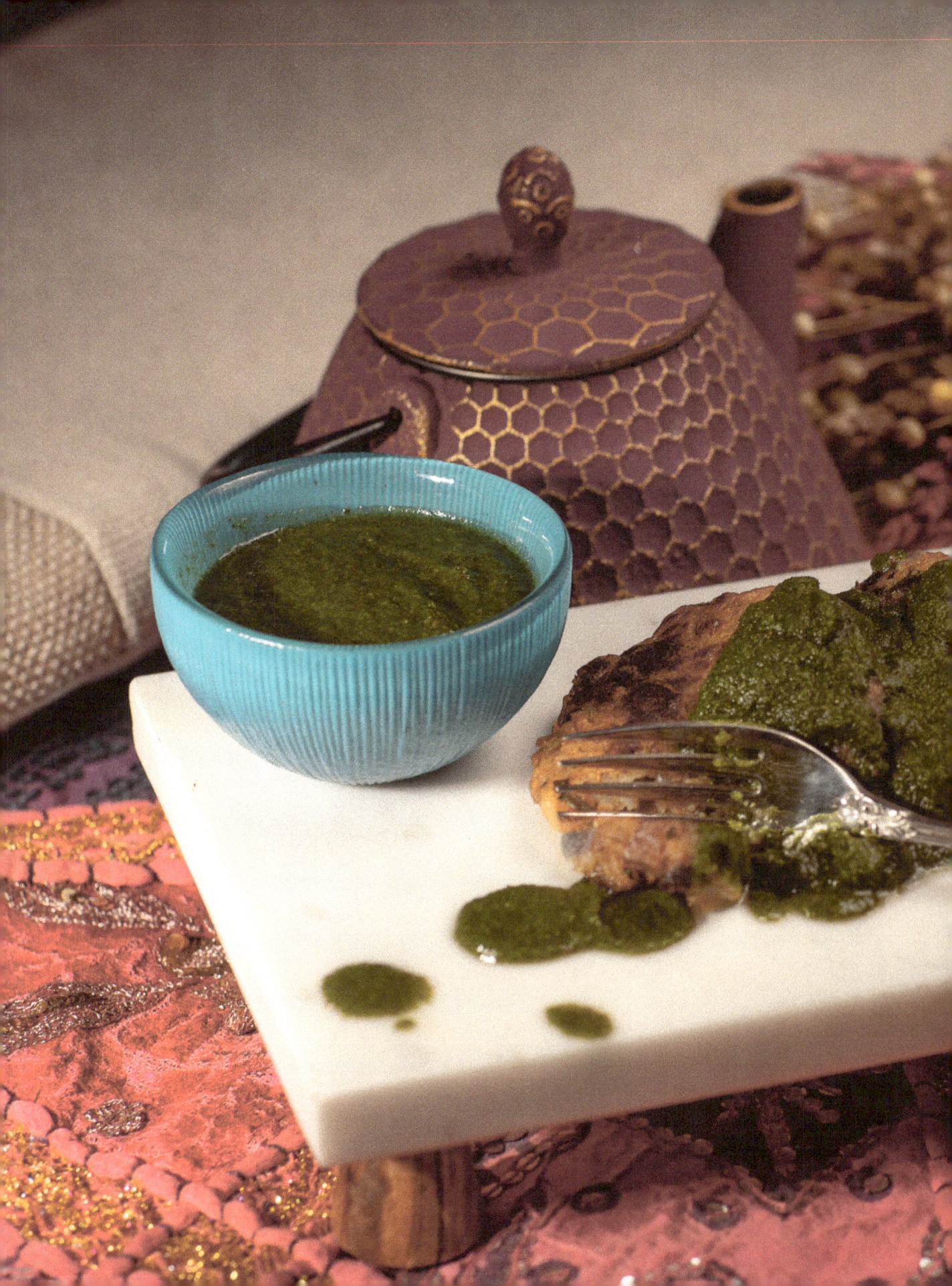

fresh start
mint chutney

As you explore these recipes, you'll notice they're more than just instructions, they're invitations. Invitations to pause, to get curious, to create with heart. The textures, the colors, the scents rising from a simmering pot—each moment is a chance to be present, to nourish not only your body, but your spirit.

Herb-packed and digestion-boosting—your go-to dressing! Crushing fresh mint and cilantro in my kitchen always brings back the scent of summer—cool, zesty, and made with love, just like mom used to serve with every meal. Who knew a handful of mint and cilantro could work such magic? This zesty green wonder is like a garden party for your taste buds—with health perks to match.

fresh start mint chutney

Mint chutney, also known as pudina chutney, is a spicy, flavorful, and healthy Indian side dip. It's a versatile condiment that adds a refreshing zing to meals, making it an ideal accompaniment for snacks, appetizers, sandwiches and wraps, grilled meats and vegetables, salads, burritos.

ingredients

2 cups chopped cilantro *(approximately 1 large bunch)*
1 cup chopped mint *(pudina)*
1/2 cup chopped red onion
6-8 tbsp of fresh lemon juice
1 1/2 tsp of chopped fresh ginger
1 tsp chopped green chilies *(optional)*
1/4 tsp red pepper chili flakes *(optional)*
Salt according to taste

directions

In a blender, add the cilantro leaves and mint. Be sure to remove the hard stems from the mint, though the softer stems can be included for added flavor. Ensure both herbs are washed thoroughly.

Include ginger, onion, salt, and lemon juice in the blender. You can choose to add either green chilies or red pepper chili flakes for heat.

Blend everything together until it is smooth.

After reaching your desired consistency, transfer the chutney to a bowl or jar. For the best flavor, it is recommended to chill the chutney thoroughly before using it. This allows the flavors to develop even further and enhances the overall taste. Enjoy your fresh and zesty chutney!

Homemade mint chutney will stay fresh in the refrigerator for up to 4 days when stored in a sealed container. You can also freeze the chutney for later use, ensuring you always have a tasty and aromatic condiment ready whenever you need it!

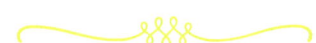

This vibrant, herb-packed chutney is full of flavor, featuring fresh mint, chilies, ginger, and garlic. It takes only 5 minutes to prepare using a blender or food processor. Plus, it's naturally gluten-free and easily customizable for a vegan diet!

a fresh detox!

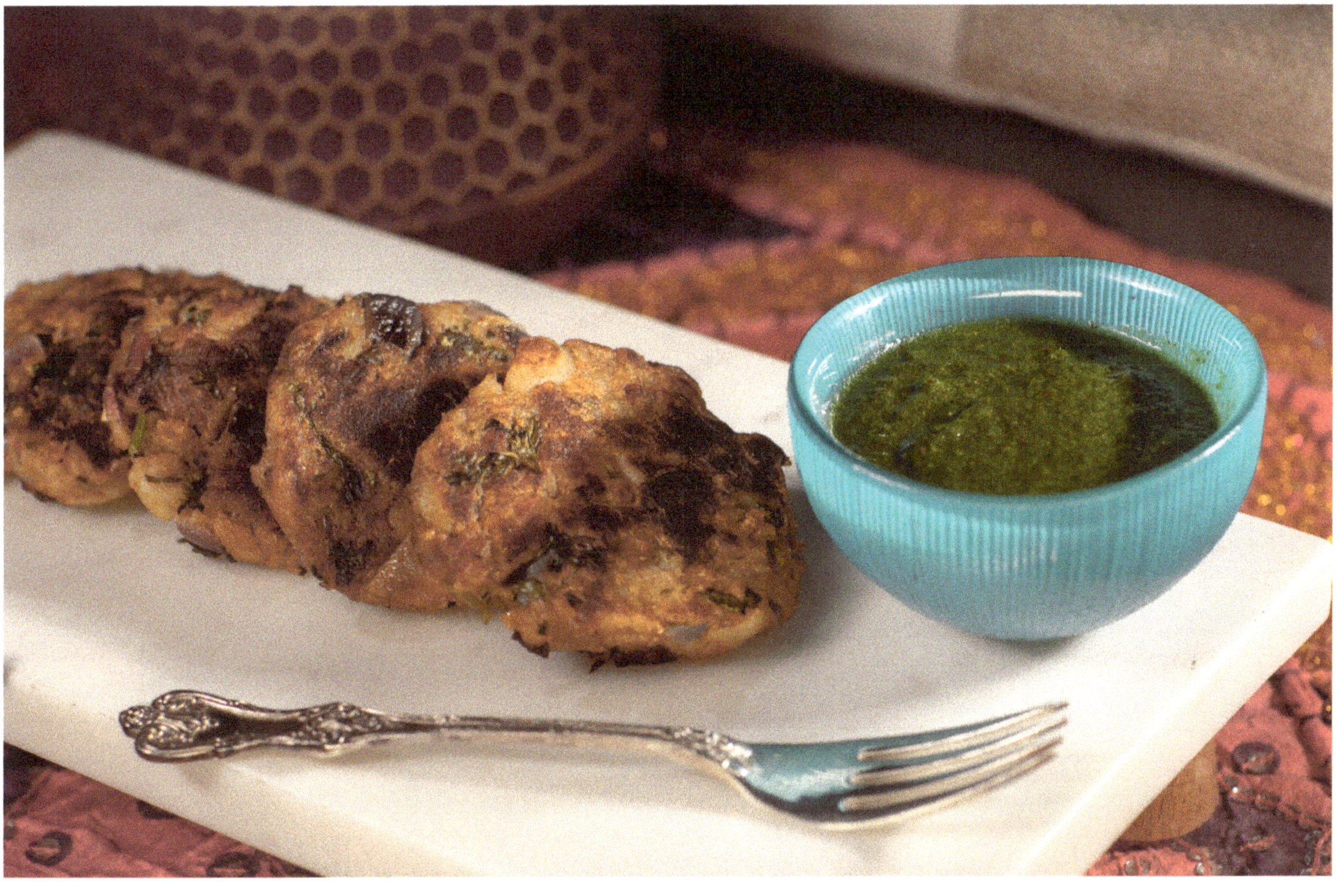

Mint has natural detoxifying properties, helping to cleanse the body and support healthy digestion. With ingredients like cilantro and lime, this chutney is full of vitamin C to support your immune system.

health benefits of the ingredients

mint

It is packed with nutrients like antioxidants, vitamin C, and fiber. It helps with digestion and activates the digestive tract. The aroma of pudina chutney also stimulates the salivary glands, which secrete digestive enzymes. Mint's antiseptic and antipruritic properties can soothe and cleanse the skin and help with acne. Mint's anti-inflammatory properties can help reduce inflammation in the stomach.

cilantro stems pack a vitamin c punch!

Did you know the stems of cilantro are rich in vitamin C? Don't throw them away—use them to boost your immune system and add extra flavor to your dishes! Packed with vitamins A, K, and C, this herb strengthens your immune system, fights oxidative stress, and helps lower blood sugar levels. Rich in antioxidants, it also supports healthy weight management.

ginger

Packed with beneficial compounds, ginger is rich in gingerol, known for its anti-inflammatory and antioxidant properties. It also contains vitamins C and B6, supporting metabolism and immune function, while its fiber content aids digestion and promotes gut health.

lemon juice

Lemon juice offers a variety of health benefits due to its high nutritional profile. It is packed with vitamin C, supporting immune health, skin, and wound healing. It contains antioxidants that help protect the body from oxidative stress and reduce inflammation. Adding lemon juice to water not only enhances the flavor but also encourages hydration. Lemon juice may aid in weight loss by promoting feelings of fullness and reducing calorie intake.

green chilies or red pepper chili flakes

Consuming chilies or red pepper flakes can provide numerous health benefits, thanks to their rich content of vitamins, minerals, and capsaicin. Spices like these are packed with vitamin C, which boosts the immune system. They also help lower LDL cholesterol, reduce inflammation, and enhance circulation, promoting better heart health.

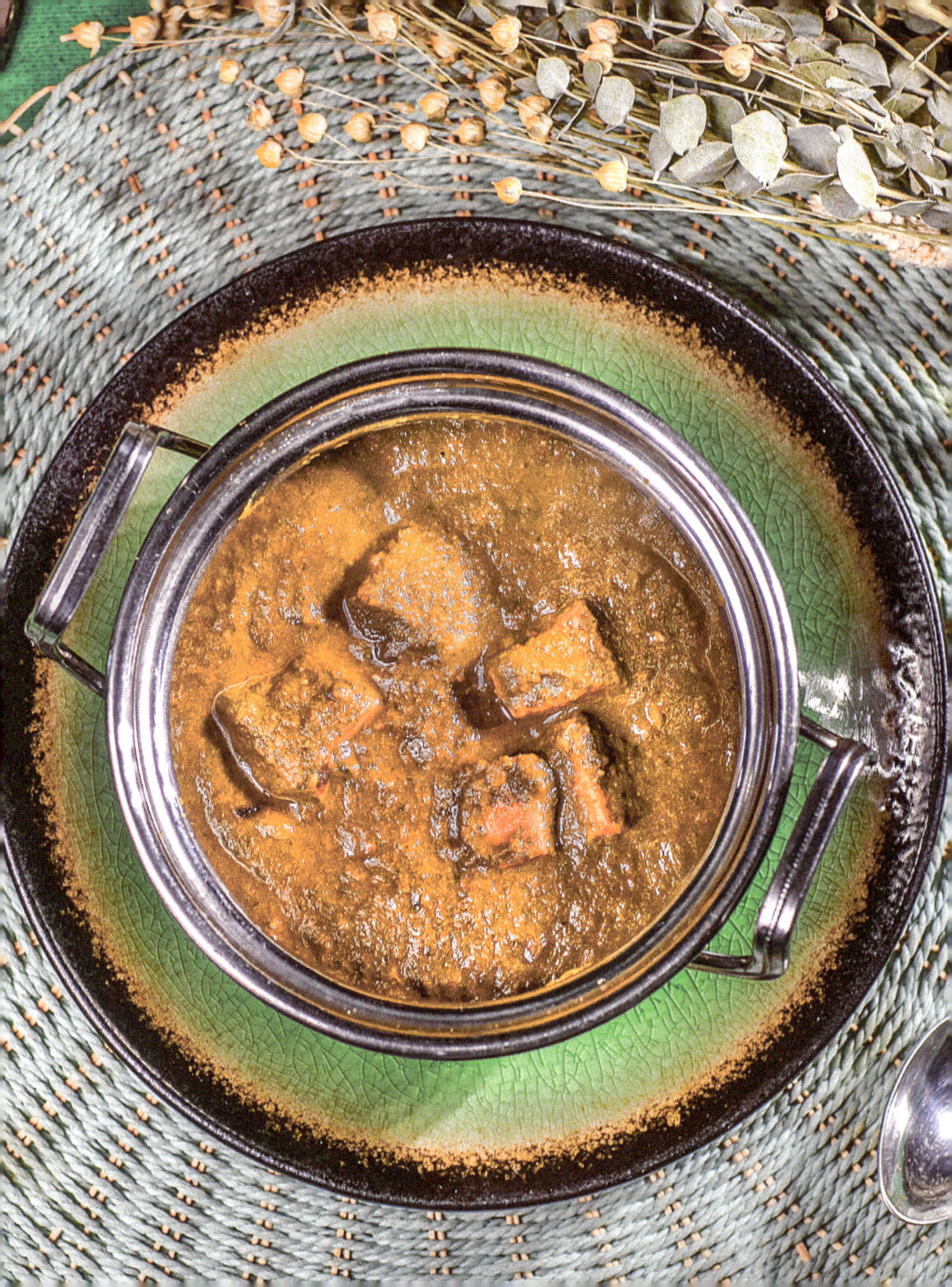

spinach paneer bliss curry (palak paneer)

In my kitchen, the most ordinary ingredients—like a handful of fresh spinach, a scoop of warm lentils, or a sprinkle of earthy spices—transform into something extraordinary.

Spinach + paneer = powerhouse combo for strength and immunity. Kid-Approved Healthy Vibes- We called it 'green cheese curry' growing up—easy to love, hard to resist, and secretly full of everything growing bodies need.

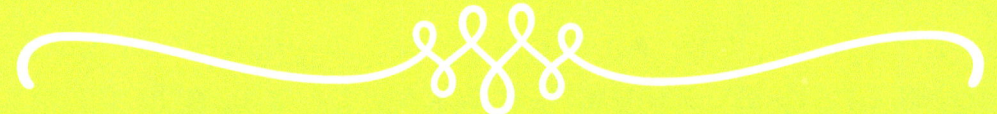

creamy without the cream

This curry gets its richness from pureed spinach and spices—no heavy cream needed. Just wholesome, heart-loving ingredients!

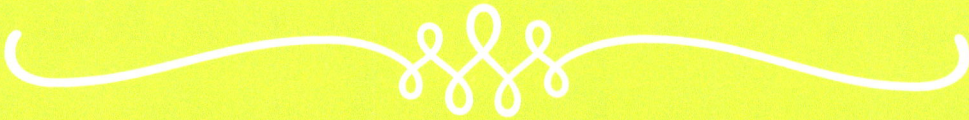

spinach paneer bliss curry (palak paneer)

Spinach with paneer curry, also known as palak paneer, is a delicious and healthy vegetarian Indian dish made with pureed spinach and Indian cottage cheese (paneer). This homemade palak paneer can be prepared in just 30-35 minutes. Serve it with any Indian bread or plain basmati rice for a truly satisfying meal!

ingredients

1 (11oz) bag of baby spinach
1 (8 oz) pack of paneer, cubed *(found in Indian grocery stores)*
2 cups finely chopped red onion
2 cups finely chopped tomatoes
3 1/2 tbsp of cooking oil *(your choice)*
1 tbsp ghee or vegan butter
1 tbsp minced garlic
2 tsp crushed fresh ginger
2 dried red chilies *(optional)*
1 tsp cumin seeds
1/2 tsp red chili powder *(adjust to taste)*
1/4 tsp turmeric powder
1/4 tsp cumin powder
1/4 tsp garam masala
Salt according to taste

directions

Wash the spinach and set it aside.

Heat oil in a pan over medium heat. Add cumin seeds and dried red chilies and sauté for a few seconds, until the seeds release their fragrance.

Add chopped garlic and sauté for few seconds.

Stir in the chopped onions and cook until they start to turn golden brown.

Add the chopped tomatoes, ginger, and salt. Mix well and cover the pan. Cook for approximately 5 minutes until the tomatoes become mushy, then add the spinach and sauté for a few minutes.

Let the mixture cool down for a few minutes and then transfer to the food processor and blend it until smooth.

Heat 2 tablespoons of oil in a separate pan and gently sauté the paneer cubes until they turn golden brown. Afterward, transfer the cubes to a bowl of warm water to keep them soft. Return the pureed spinach mixture to the same pan and add turmeric powder, red chili powder, and cumin powder. Sauté for 7-8 minutes on low heat.

Add garam masala and butter, mix everything well, and cook for about 8-10 minutes.

Cover the pan, turn off the heat, and let it sit for at least 5 minutes before serving. Serve hot with roti, naan, paratha, or rice.

Enjoy your delicious spinach paneer curry!

Palak paneer is a classic North Indian dish and a popular choice in Indian households. Its rich, creamy spinach base paired with tender paneer cubes makes it a comforting and nutritious delight. It's magical.

Let's dive into why Palak Paneer is such a fantastic dish to add to your meal rotation:

I love this recipe! Palak Paneer is truly a powerhouse of nutrients, offering a balance of protein, iron, vitamins, and antioxidants. It is not only a delicious way to enjoy spinach and paneer, but it is also a fantastic option for supporting overall health, from boosting immunity to supporting digestion and heart health. The combination of flavors and health benefits makes it an amazing addition to any meal plan.

rich in iron
The spinach (palak) is an excellent source of iron, which is crucial for healthy blood circulation and preventing anemia.

helps with weight management
The high fiber and protein content in Palak Paneer help you feel full for longer, supporting appetite control and weight management.

supports bone health
Both spinach and paneer are rich in calcium, which helps in strengthening bones and teeth.

high in protein
Paneer is a great source of protein, which is essential for muscle repair, growth, and overall body function.

aids digestion
The high fiber content in spinach promotes healthy digestion and regular bowel movements.

boosts immunity
Spinach is packed with vitamins A and C, which help in boosting the immune system and fighting off infections.

rich in antioxidants
Spinach contains antioxidants like lutein and zeaxanthin, which support eye health and reduce oxidative stress in the body.

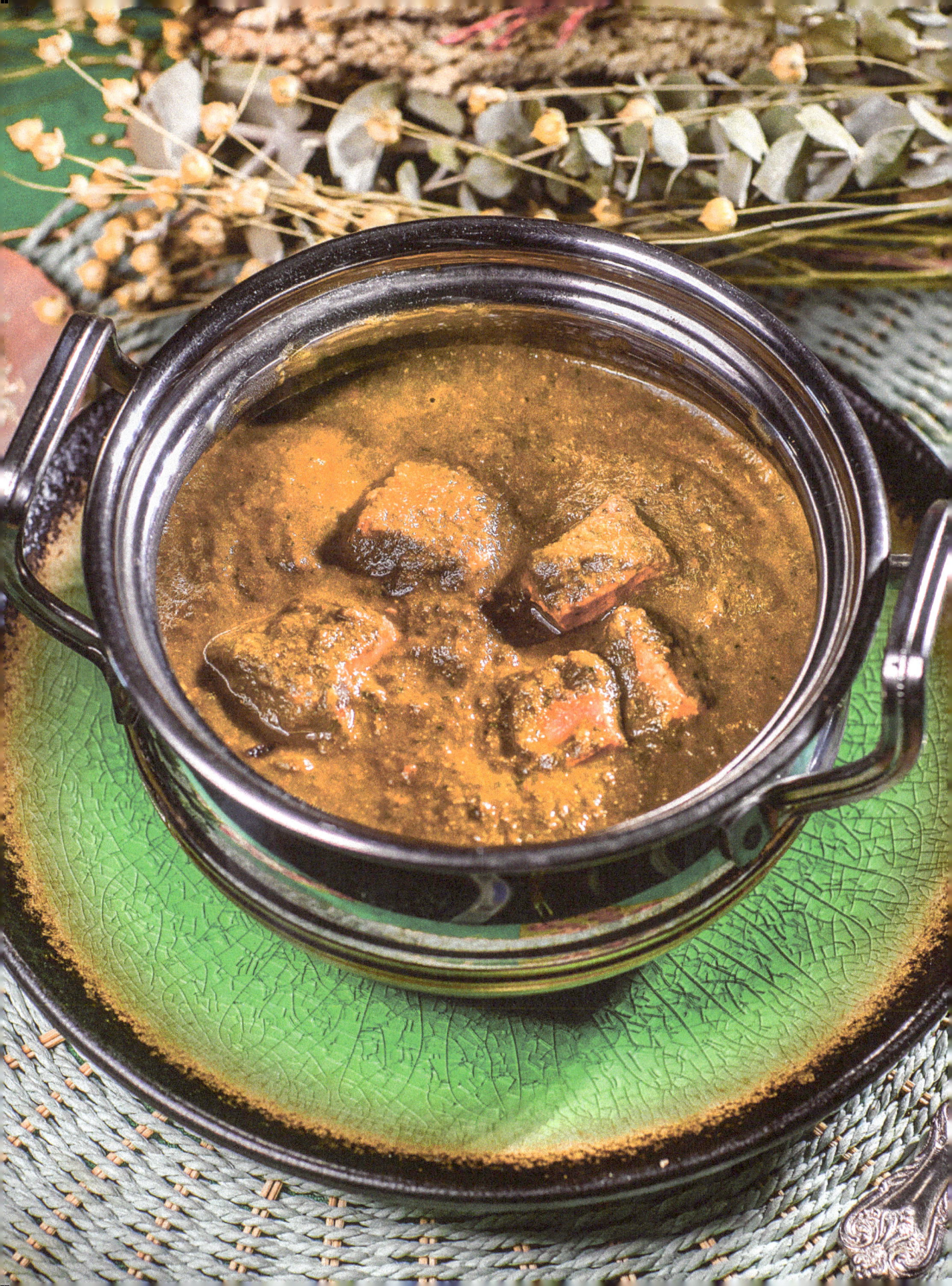

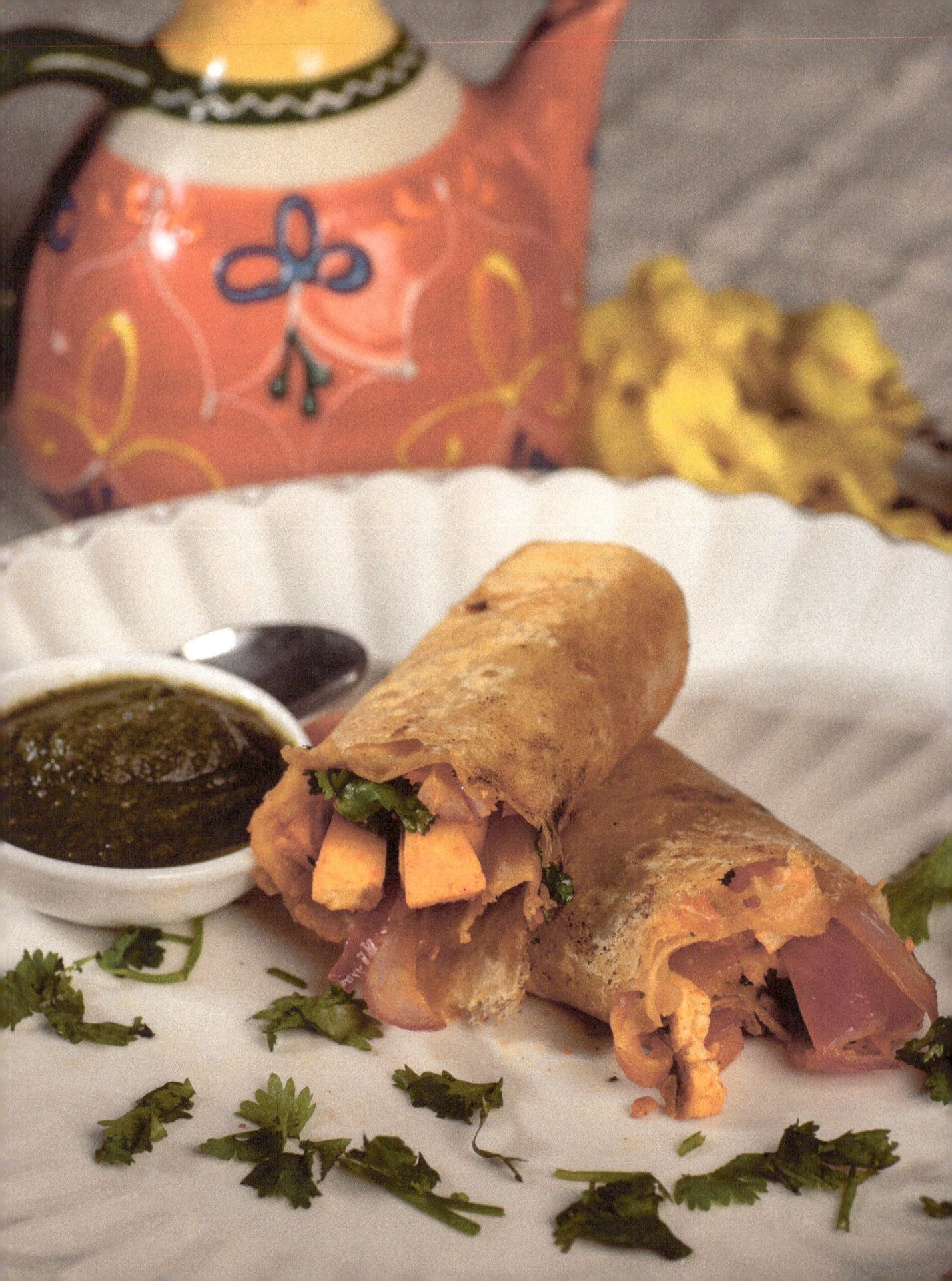

wrap-tastic paneer kathi roll

This book was created for families like mine—where meals are shared, laughter is loud, and food is a love language. Whether you're a teenager discovering your way in the kitchen or an adult looking for fresh inspiration, you'll find something here that satisfies both your cravings and your curiosity.

Bold flavors, handheld style. Fuel up with flavorful paneer wrapped in a whole grain embrace.

wrap-tastic paneer kathi roll

A Paneer Kathi Roll is a delicious Indian wrap. Kathi Roll is one of India's most popular grab-and-go street foods. I enjoy this quick vegetarian version that uses zesty paneer cubes (cottage cheese) as the main ingredient. Packed with a delightful blend of spices and flavors, this super easy dish can be prepared in under 30 minutes.

ingredients

3-4 Indian plain paratha *(store bought)*
1 1/2 cup tomatoes, thinly sliced
1 cup onion, thinly sliced
1 cup chopped lettuce
1 cup paneer thinly sliced *(Indian cheese)*
1/2 cup Greek yogurt
2-3 tbsp olive oil
2 tbsp chopped cilantro
1/4 tsp cumin powder
1/4 tsp coriander powder
1/4 tsp chili powder
1/4 tsp chopped garlic
1/4 tsp chaat masala
Salt and pepper according to taste

directions

Slice the paneer thinly and combine it with yogurt and all the spices, then let it marinate for two hours. Heat some oil in a pan, add chopped garlic, and sauté the paneer until it becomes golden brown. Then, add the onions and tomatoes to the same pan and cook for 5-7 minutes, or until they become crispy. You can use any brand of plain paratha. If you are using frozen ones, I recommend taking them out a few hours before preparing the recipe to thaw them. Then, heat them in a pan before filling with paneer and veggies. If you have fresh paratha, which some stores offer, you can simply heat it on a griddle for a few minutes. In a separate pan, spray some oil and cook the paratha. Spread mint chutney on the paratha, then layer with the paneer and veggies, and sprinkle with chaat masala. Roll it up like a burrito and cut it in half. Enjoy your delicious Indian kathi roll!

This recipe is packed with flavor, easy to make, and ideal for serving a crowd! It serves 4 people.

For Mint Chutney: Please see the recipe on page 57.

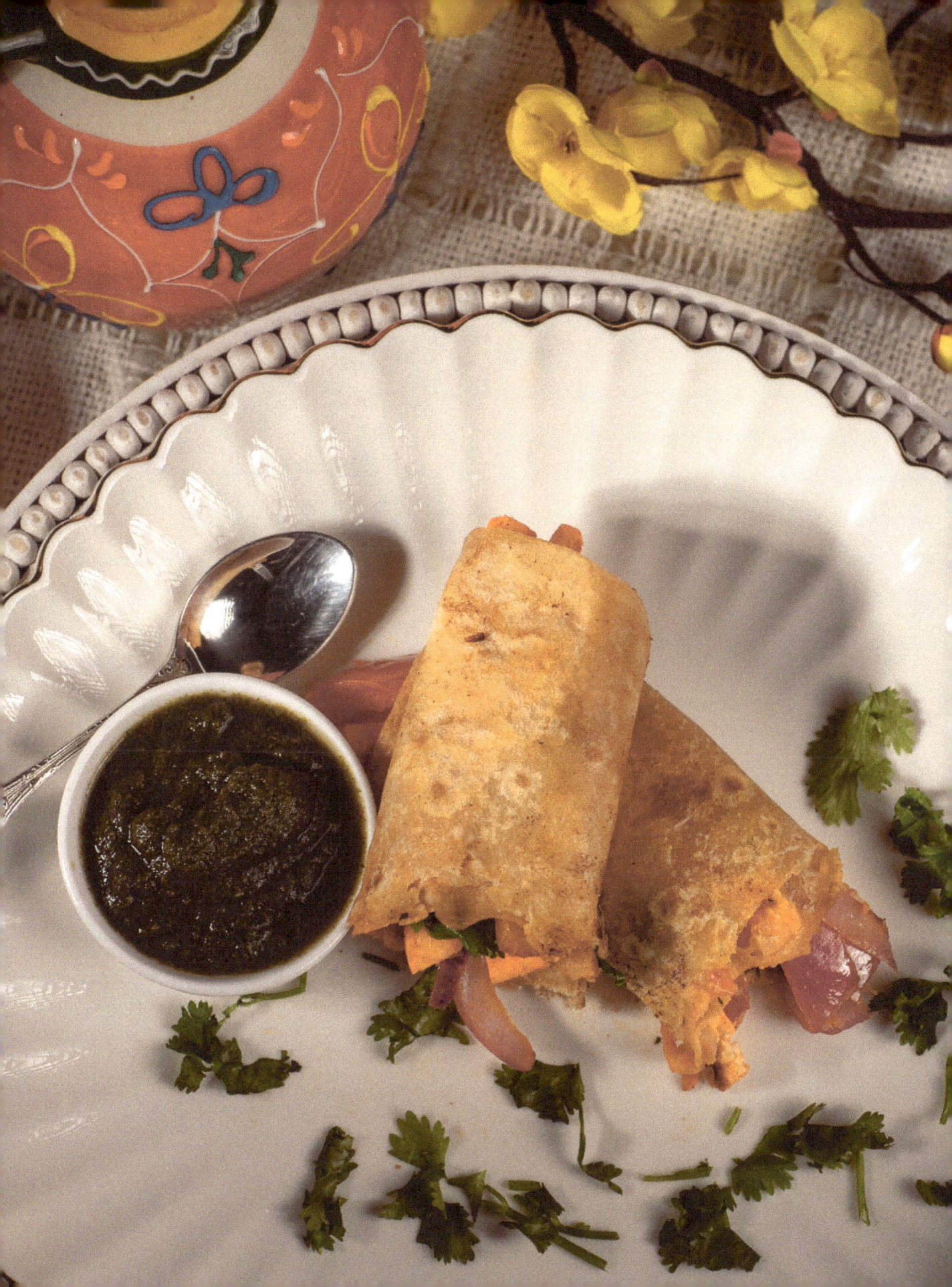

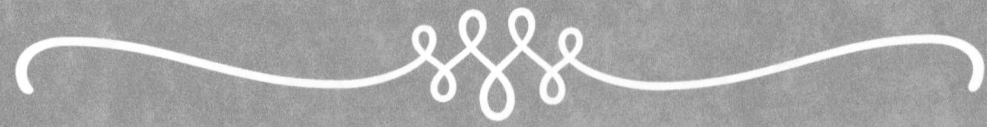

balanced meal in a wrap

A Kathi roll offers a convenient, balanced combination of proteins, healthy fats, and carbs, providing long-lasting energy while keeping hunger at bay.

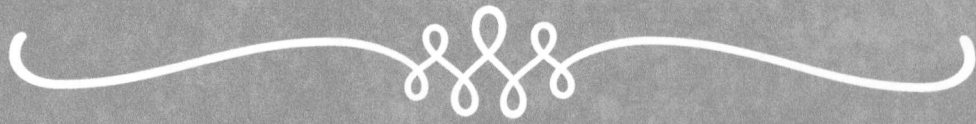

This recipe features paneer (Indian cottage cheese) marinated in yogurt and aromatic spices, cooked with vegetables, topped with tangy mint chutney, and then wrapped in a crispy paratha. A paratha is a type of Indian flatbread that is typically made with whole wheat flour and cooked on a flat griddle, or tava, with a small amount of oil or ghee. It is a delicious roll that will appeal to both vegetarians and meat lovers!

I would like to discuss the health benefits of paneer. Paneer is a staple ingredient in Indian cuisine. Paneer offers several health benefits, making it a great addition to a balanced diet:

high in protein

Paneer is an excellent source of protein, especially for vegetarians.

rich in calcium

Paneer is a good source of calcium, which is vital for healthy bones and teeth, and can help prevent osteoporosis.

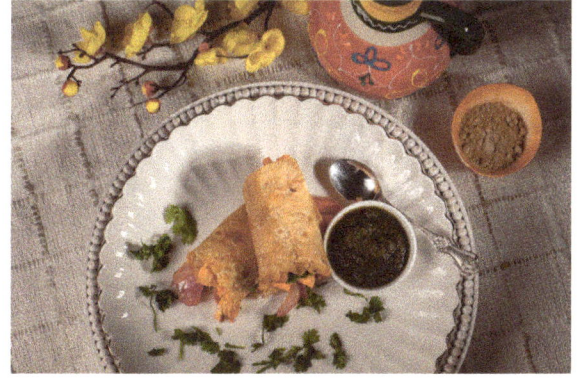

boosts digestion

The probiotics in paneer (especially homemade or fermented varieties) can promote a healthy gut and improve digestion.

rich in vitamins

Paneer is a source of essential vitamins, including vitamin B12, which is important for energy production, and vitamin A, which supports skin and eye health.

supports immune function

Paneer contains various micronutrients like zinc and magnesium that contribute to a strong immune system.

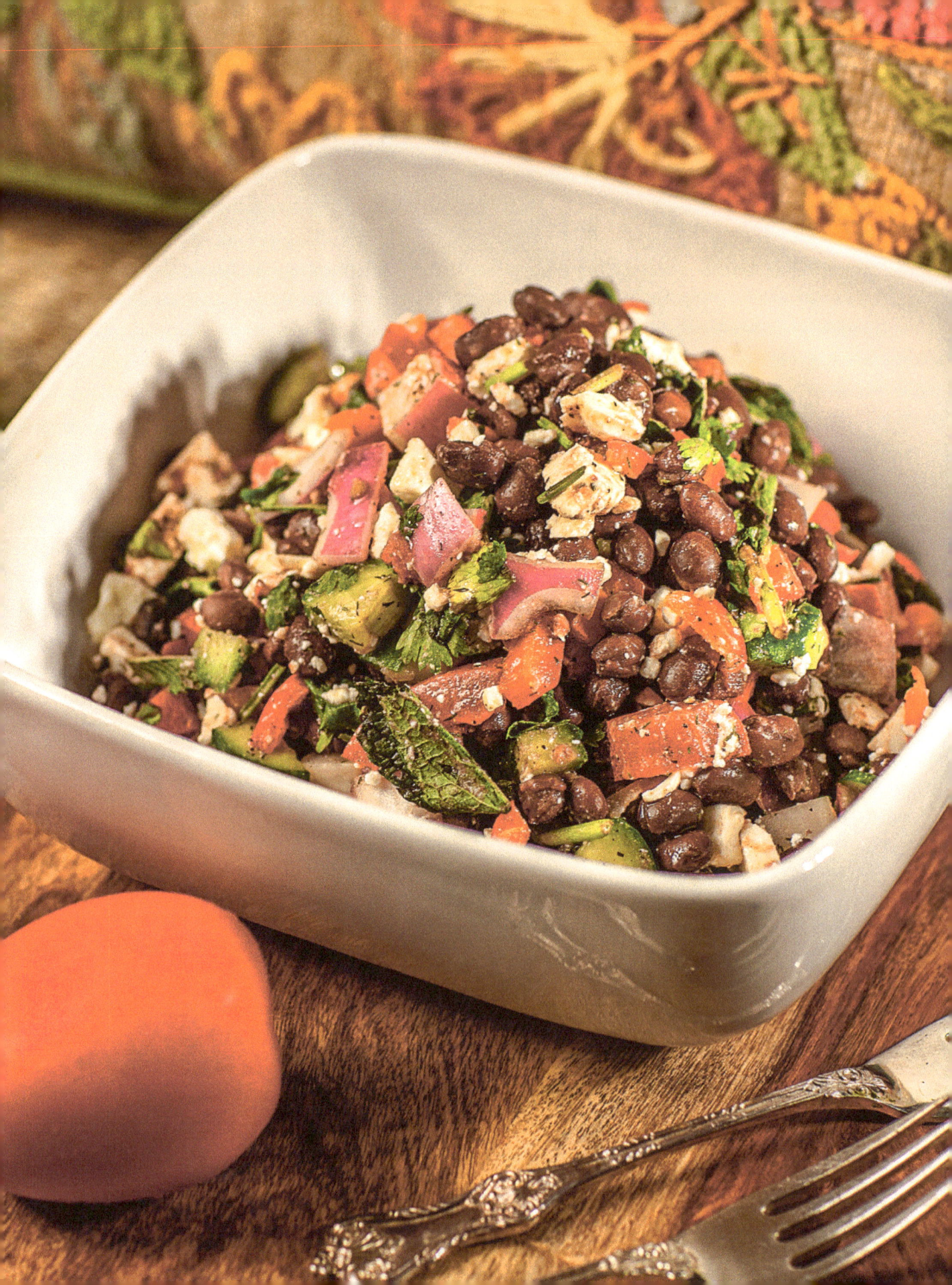

protein-packed mediterranean bean delight

Food isn't about strict rules or boring healthy food. It's about flavor-packed dishes that celebrate wellness and joy in every bite. From protein-rich meals that keep you energized through long school or workdays, to fiber-filled snacks that actually taste fun, every recipe is a balance of taste, texture, and nutrients.

This salad is like a burst of sunshine on your plate! Full of vibrant colors, fresh herbs, and hearty beans, it's the perfect dish to accompany a rich meal or serve as a refreshing main on a warm day. A refreshing, fiber-rich salad with protein and crunch.

protein-packed mediterranean bean delight

I absolutely love Mediterranean-style salads—they are refreshing, flavorful, and endlessly satisfying. This Mediterranean black bean salad is no exception; the combination of ingredients makes every bite a delight! This salad brings together fresh produce and simple pantry staples for a vibrant and satisfying dish.

ingredients

2 cans black beans, rinsed and drained
1 cup chopped red bell pepper
1 cup chopped baby cucumbers
1/2 cup chopped red onions
1/2 cup chopped Roma tomatoes
1/2 cup diced red radish
1/4 cup feta cheese
5-6 tbsp red wine vinegar
3/4 tbsp fresh mint leaves
3/4 tbsp cilantro
1 1/2 tsp diced pickled jalapeno pepper
1 tsp dried dill
1 tsp dried basil
Salt and pepper according to taste

directions

This recipe is super easy to throw together once everything is chopped and diced.

In a large bowl, combine the drained black beans, diced red onion, cucumber, radish, red bell pepper, tomatoes, jalapeño, and crumbled feta cheese.

Add the fresh and dried herbs, salt, and pepper followed by red wine vinegar.

Gently toss everything together, ensuring the dressing and ingredients are evenly mixed.

Cover and refrigerate for at least 30 minutes to let the flavors meld beautifully. Serve chilled—and enjoy every bite!

storing the salad

Store any leftover Mediterranean black bean salad in an airtight container in the fridge for up to 3 days.

tiny beans, big impact

Just 1/2 cup of beans provides nearly a third of your daily fiber needs—and that means better blood sugar balance and energy.

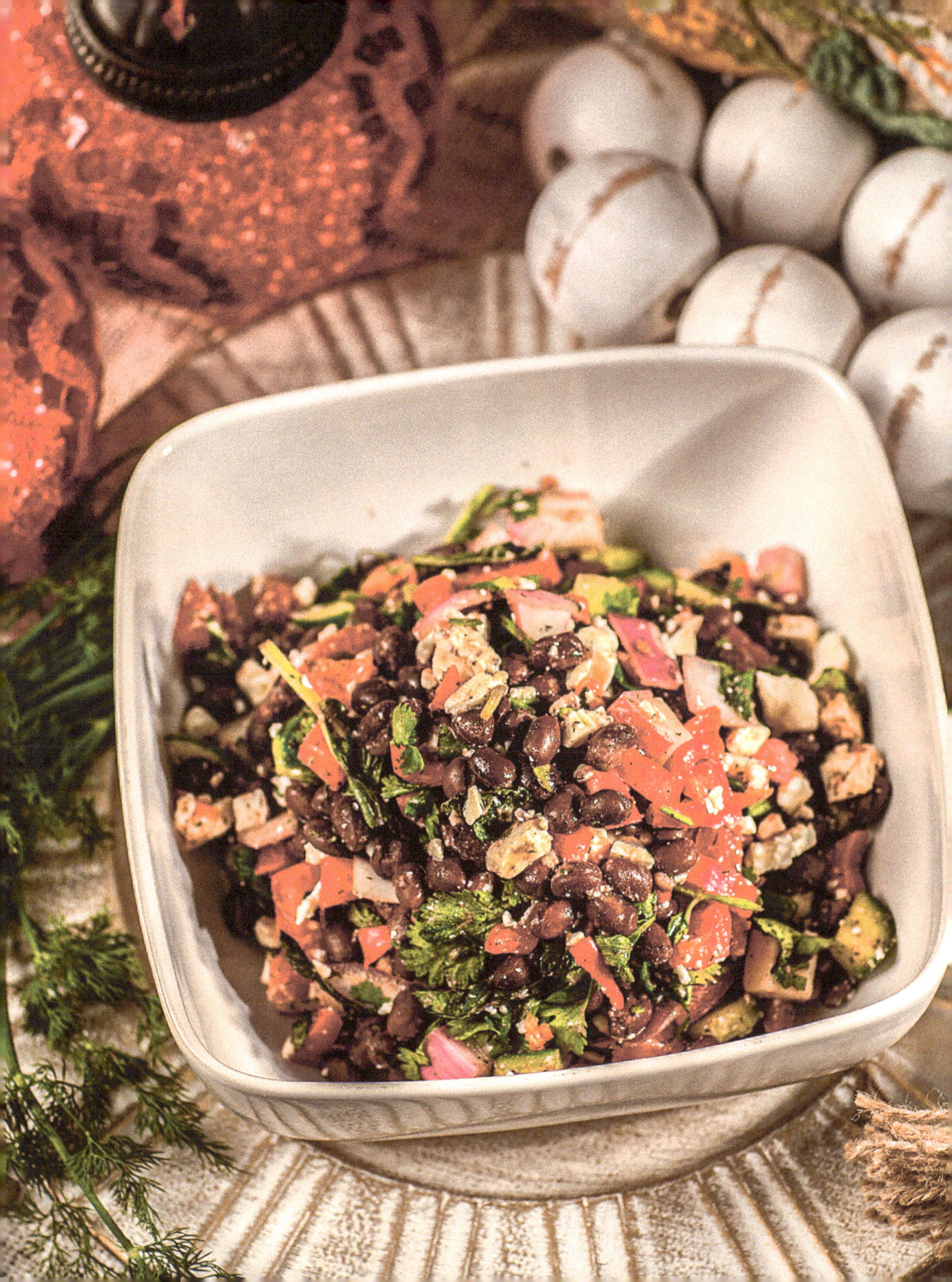

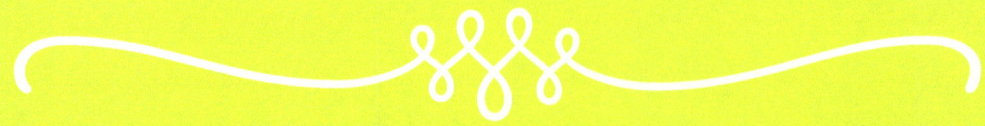

tiny beans, big impact

Just 1/2 cup of beans provides nearly a third of your daily fiber needs—and that means better blood sugar balances and energy.

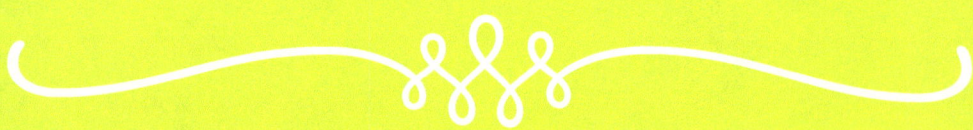

why this salad is a smart choice

I call this salad a harmony of wholesome ingredients. This salad is my go-to for those busy days when we need a meal that's both quick and nourishing. Packed with fiber, protein, and healthy fats, it's the kind of dish that makes everyone feel good from the inside out. It's a reminder that even a simple, vibrant salad can support a healthy lifestyle while tasting absolutely delightful! Healthy never tasted this fun! This vibrant Mediterranean bean salad is loaded with **fiber, plant-based protein, and heart-healthy fats.** Black beans help you feel full and energized, while the mix of fresh veggies adds **vitamins, minerals,** and a refreshing crunch. Feta cheese offers a touch of **calcium**, and herbs bring heart-healthy goodness. It's a colorful, feel-good dish that is as nourishing as it is tasty

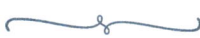

This Mediterranean-style salad is perfect for spring picnics, summer potlucks, or cozy fall gatherings. It's a crowd-pleasing side dish that fits most special diets—even vegetarian and gluten-free.

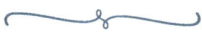

It comes together in just about 20 minutes with a simple chop, whisk, and toss. Quick, fresh, and flavorful, I hope it becomes a go-to recipe in your kitchen too!

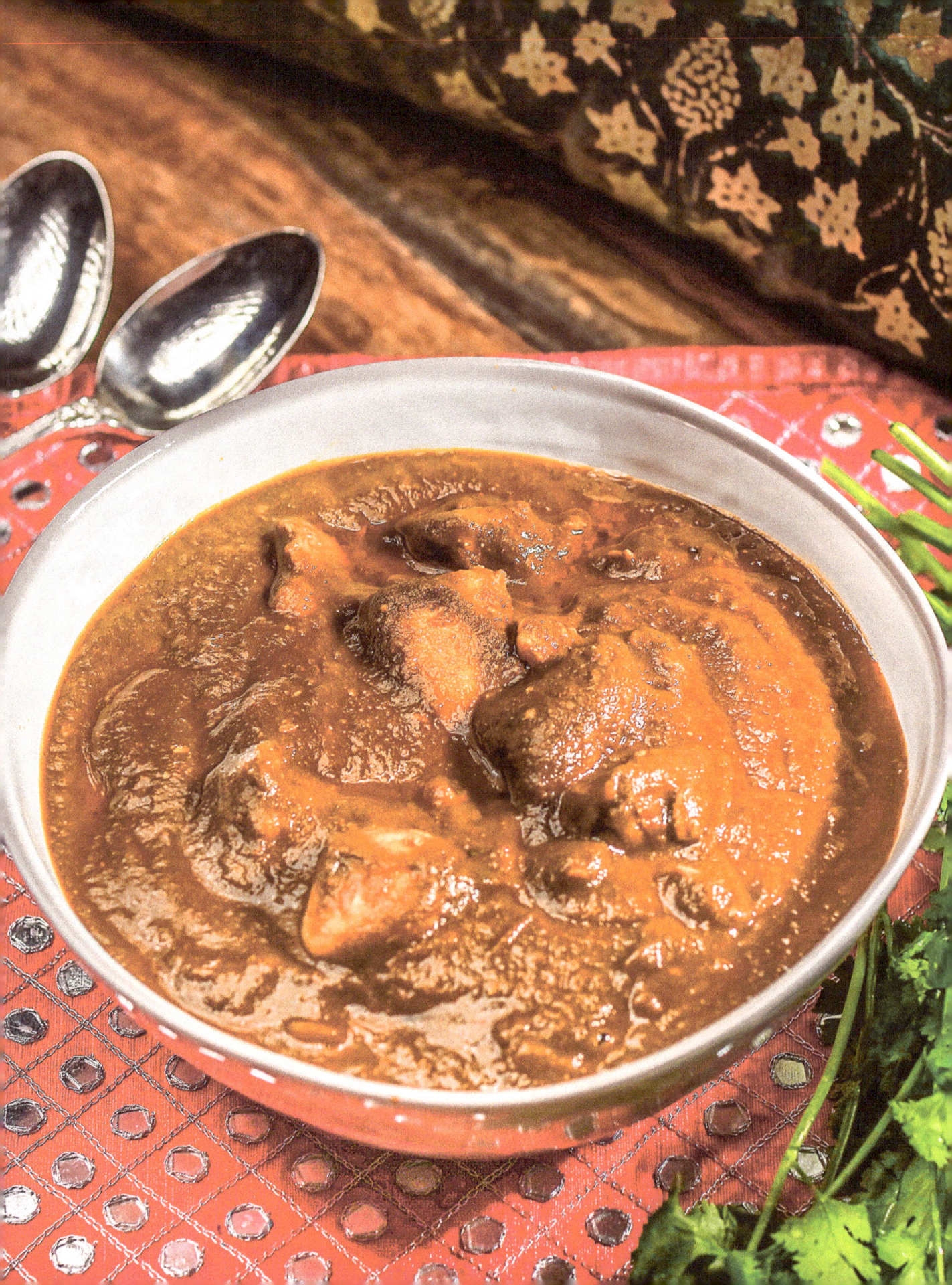

palak infused chicken

In every recipe, I've poured my passion for using simple, nutrient-rich ingredients that nourish the body and comfort the soul. I've always believed that the best meals don't come from fancy techniques or expensive ingredients, but from the care we pour into choosing what nourishes us.

A creamy, spiced spinach and chicken combo loaded with essential nutrients. The marriage of tender chicken and vibrant spinach in this dish is one of my favorites. It's not just healthy, it's a comforting, hearty meal that feels like a warm hug from the inside.

palak infused chicken

Palak Chicken is a flavorful Indian dish that combines tender chicken pieces with a spiced spinach gravy. This dish, rooted in North Indian cuisine, is enriched with aromatic spices like cumin, coriander, garam masala, and kasthuri methi, creating a deliciously fragrant experience. Whether paired with fluffy basmati rice, tucked into warm roti, or enjoyed straight from the bowl, this dish hits the sweet spot between health and flavor.

ingredients

1 1/2 lbs cubed chicken thighs, boneless
5 cups baby spinach
1 cup chopped onions
1 cup tomato puree
1/2 cup chopped Roma tomatoes
3 tbsp olive oil
1 tbsp coriander powder
1 tbsp cumin powder
1 tsp dried fenugreek leaves (kasthuri methi)
1/2 tsp crushed fresh ginger
1/2 tsp crushed garlic
1/2 tsp red chili powder (Kashmiri)- or according to taste
1/2 tsp garam masala
3 bay leaves
Salt according to taste
Water as needed

directions

Heat oil in a large pan over low to medium heat, add cumin seeds and bay leaves, and sauté briefly. Add cubed chicken, cooking for a few minutes before incorporating all dry spices except garam masala. Continue to cook the chicken with the spices for 8-10 minutes until it reaches a golden-brown color. Set it aside.

In the same pan heat oil in a pan over medium heat. Once hot, add crushed ginger and garlic, and sauté for a few minutes until fragrant. Add chopped onions and cook until they turn golden brown. Then, incorporate chopped tomatoes and cook until they release their moisture.

Add the spinach to the pan and cook until it wilts. Allow the mixture to cool, then transfer it to a blender and blend until it reaches a moderately thick consistency, avoiding over-blending to maintain some texture.

Using the same pan previously utilized for sautéing the onions and tomatoes, pour in the pureed spinach mixture along with tomato puree. Let it cook over medium-low heat for 5–8 minutes. Stir in the remaining dry spices, including garam masala, and cook for another 7–9 minutes.

Then, add the pre-cooked chicken, mix well, and let it simmer on low heat so the flavors can come together beautifully.

Pour in 1/4 cup of water, adjusting as necessary to achieve your desired consistency, since the spinach mixture may thicken. Continue cooking for a few more minutes until the oil separates, indicating that the palak chicken is ready. Serve hot with naan or any type of white rice!

I thoroughly enjoy preparing this dish due to its rich flavors and numerous health benefits. Creating a healthier version that tastes just as delightful as those made with cream or fat is entirely achievable. Plus, it is a healthy and budget-friendly meal.

This recipe is definitely worth trying. It uses a few select spices, but each one plays an important role, complementing the others perfectly. Also, this recipe doesn't have a very saucy consistency; it's a bit thicker. Palak Chicken, featuring chicken and spinach, offers a combination of protein, vitamins, and minerals, making it a healthy and flavorful meal. Enjoy this hearty dish that brings warmth and nutrition to your table!

did you know?

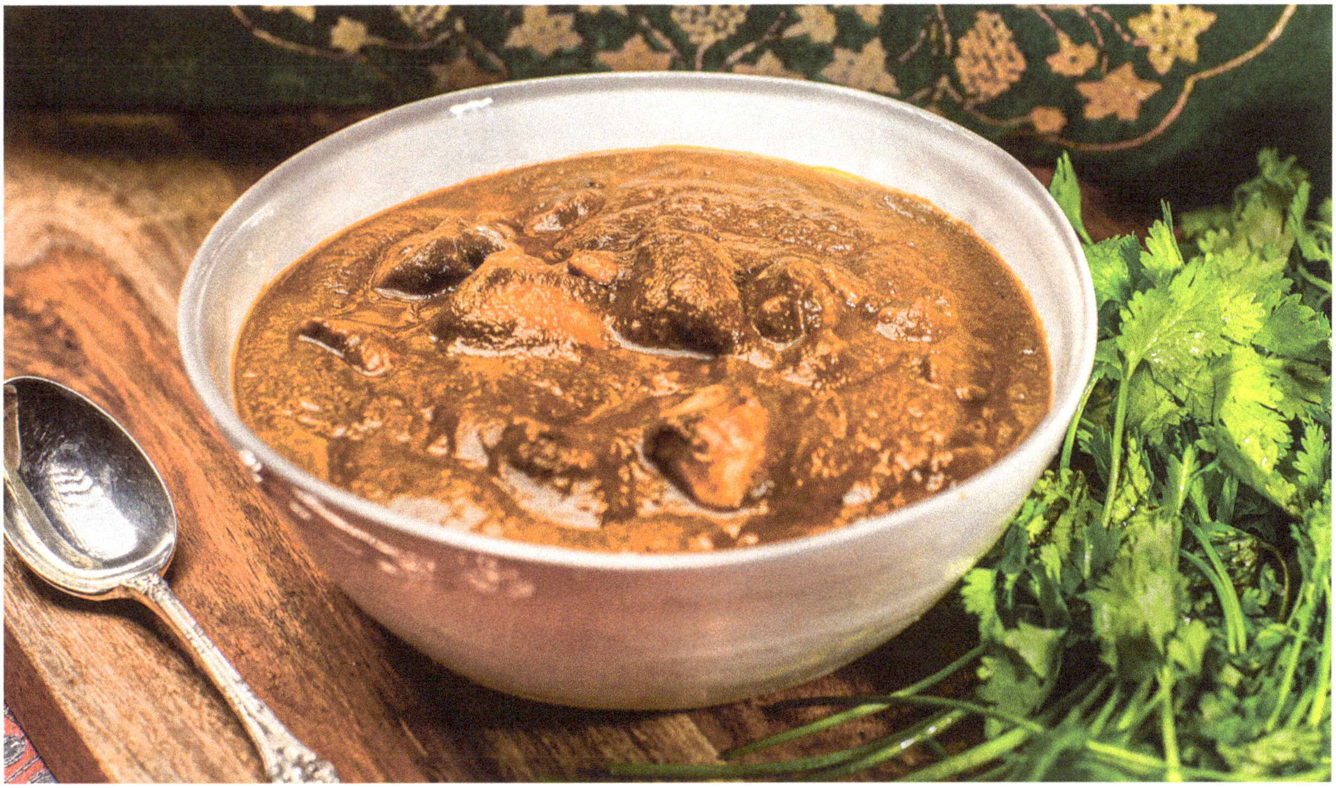

Just one cup of cooked spinach gives you more than 100% of your daily vitamin K—great for bones and healing! Spinach brings the iron, chicken brings the protein—together they are a dream team for energy, focus, and strength. Perfect after school or after sports.

Let's dive deeper into nutritional value of some of the ingredients:

spinach

Spinach, a key ingredient, is a powerhouse of vitamins and minerals, including vitamins A and C, and iron. Spinach, with its high vitamin and mineral content, can help boost immunity. Spinach is also known to promote digestion.

chicken

Chicken provides a good source of lean, high-quality protein, which is essential for building and repairing body tissues.

kasuri methi

Kasuri methi, or dried fenugreek leaves, is a flavorful addition to many dishes and offers a variety of health benefits. Incorporating this aromatic herb into your diet can contribute positively to your overall well-being. It aids in digestion, regulates blood sugar levels, and supports heart health. Additionally, kasuri methi enhances skin and hair health.

kashmiri red chili powder

In the early 20th century, the first Kashmiri chili powder was created in India by grinding dried Kashmiri Mirch into a fine powder. This powder quickly became popular among Indian chefs and was soon exported to various parts of the world. It is packed with antioxidants, provides several health benefits, including anti-inflammatory properties, enhanced digestion, and blood pressure regulation. It may help boost metabolism, potentially assisting with weight loss.

bay leaves

Bay leaves, including bay leaves in your diet, can provide various health benefits while adding flavor to your meals. They can help regulate blood sugar levels. Bay leaves are a good source of vitamins A, C, and folic acid, as well as minerals like iron, calcium, and magnesium.

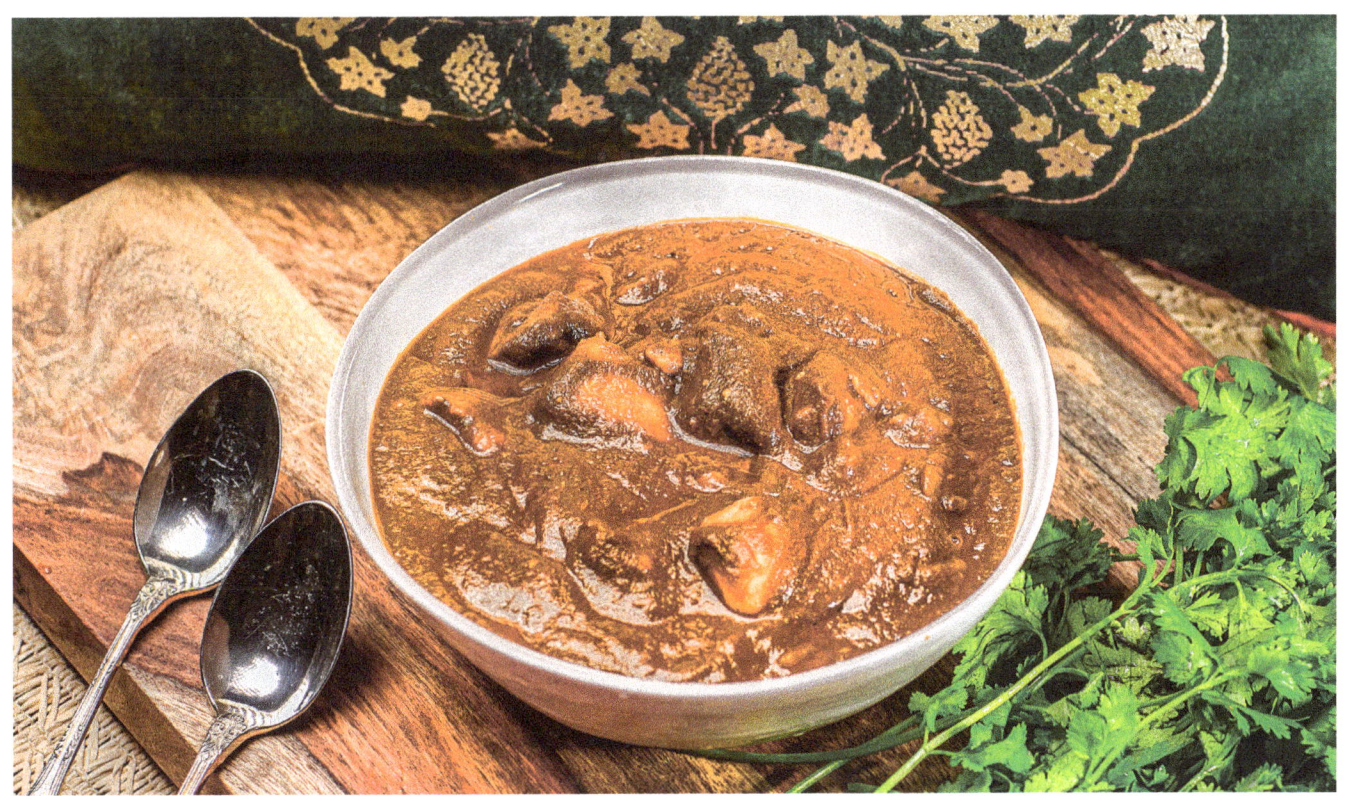

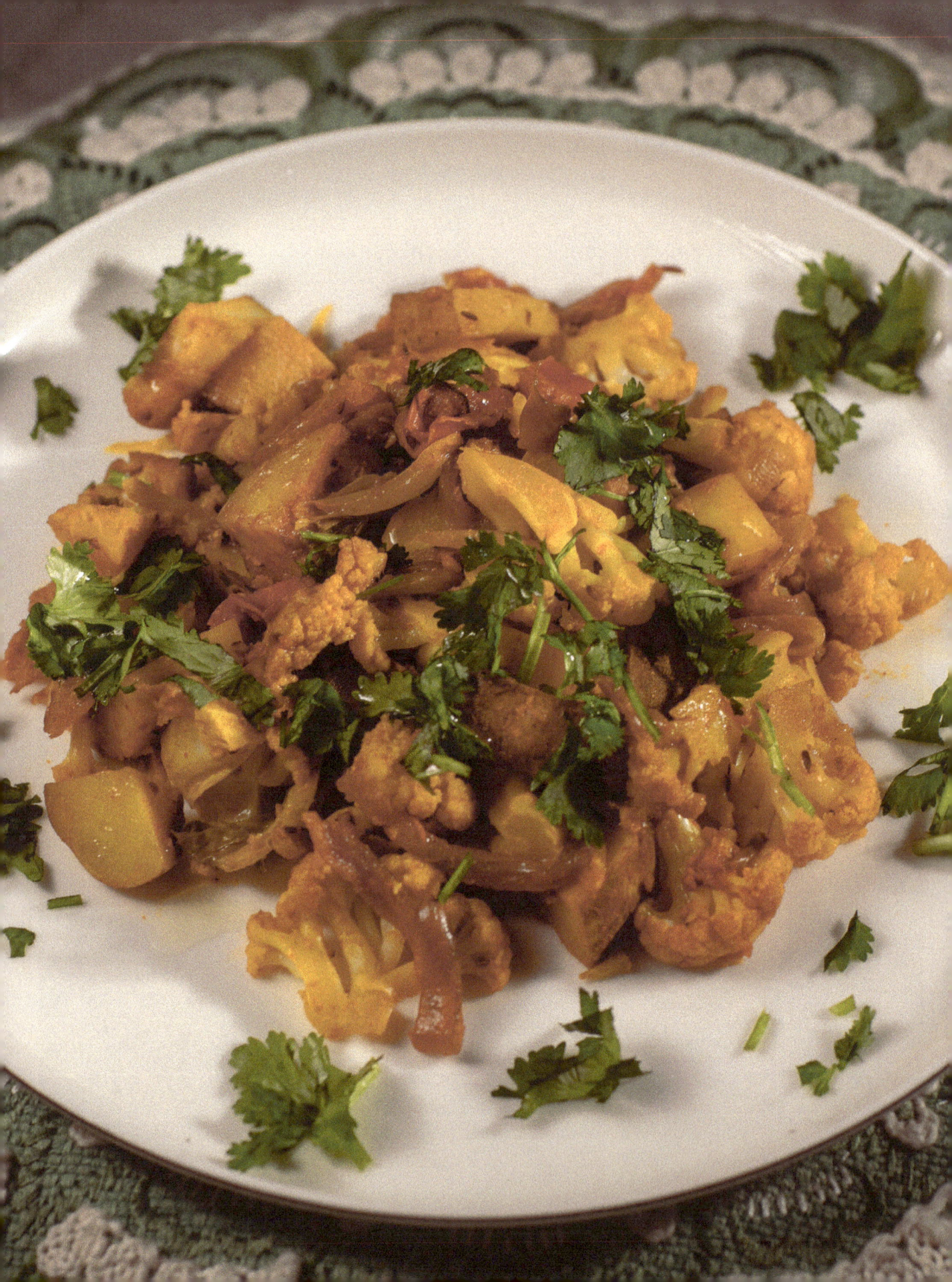

gobi aloo power bowl

Wholesome food has a quiet magic. It fills our homes with comfort, fuels our bodies with strength, and connects us to something deeper—our health, our culture, and the people we share it with. Every ingredient has a story.

A delicious simple dish that brings a big flavor with just a few ingredients. This recipe is one of those treasures that has been passed down in my family, always bringing us together.

Whether it's a weekday dinner or a special occasion, Gobi Aloo is always the star of the show! The magical blend of turmeric and cumin that turns this dish into a masterpiece.

gobi aloo power bowl

This dish is the ultimate comfort food for anyone who loves the enchanting flavors of Indian cuisine. Made with pantry staples, it is bound to steal your heart with its simplicity and delicious taste.

ingredients

2 cups chopped cauliflower florets (*1 small cauliflower*)
1 cup red potatoes, cubed
1 cup sliced red onion
1 cup of sliced tomatoes
3 tbsp chopped cilantro
2 tbsp olive oil
2 tsp minced ginger
2 tsp minced garlic
1 tsp ground cumin powder
1 tsp ground coriander powder
1/2 tsp turmeric powder
1/2 tsp cumin seeds
1/3 tsp red chili powder
1/2 tsp garam masala
Salt according to taste

directions

Heat 2 tablespoons of oil in a large pot over medium-high heat. Add cumin seeds and cook for a few seconds, allowing them to turn golden brown and begin popping. Reduce the heat to medium, then add the minced garlic and ginger, sautéing briefly until fragrant. Add the onion and cook until golden brown, then stir in the tomatoes and cover the pot, letting them cook on medium heat for 5-7 minutes. Add the spice powders—coriander, turmeric, cumin, and chili powder—and mix until well combined, cooking for another few minutes until fragrant.

Add the potatoes and cauliflower to the mixture, cover, and cook on low heat. Stir occasionally for about 10-15 minutes, until the potatoes are soft, and the cauliflower stays slightly crunchy, without becoming soggy. Add garam masala, mix well, and cook on low heat for an additional 5-7 minutes.

Cook until the vegetables are tender, then garnish with fresh cilantro.

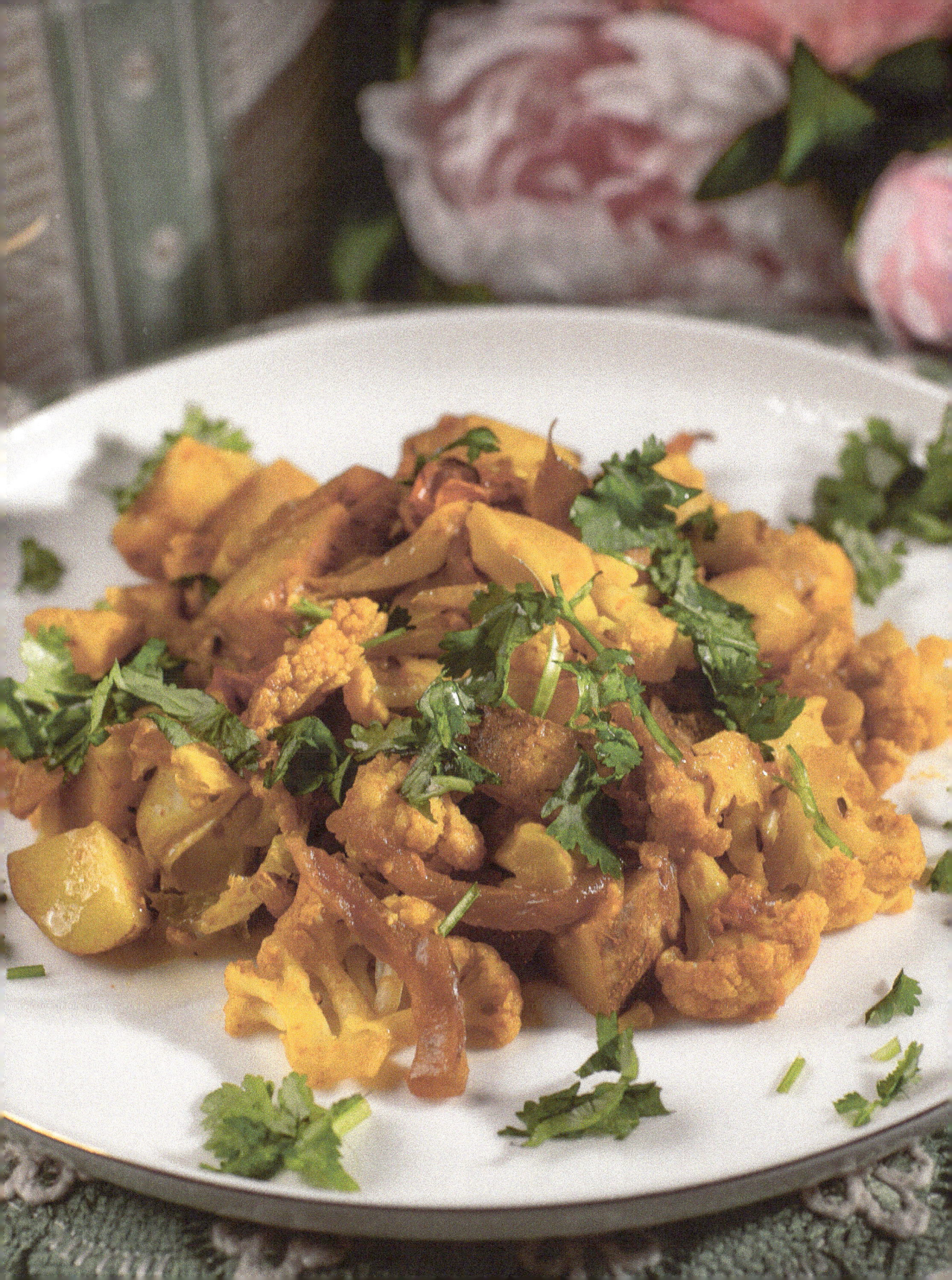

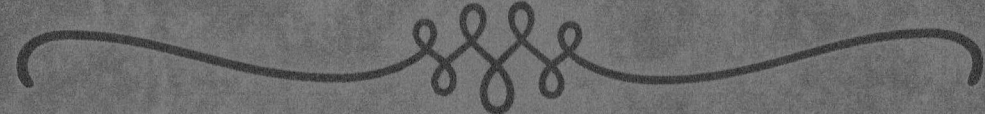

veggie power

Cauliflower is rich in fiber and antioxidants, while potatoes add potassium and vitamin C for a hearty, nutritious meal.

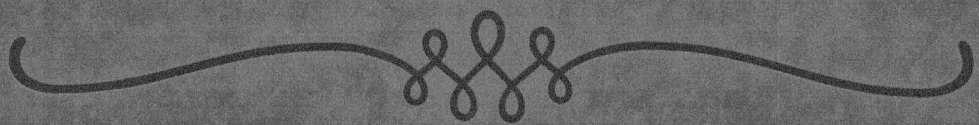

home-cooked comfort health benefits

I once asked a friend what came to mind when they thought of home-cooked Indian food, and they immediately said gobi aloo. I enjoy making this dish because it is packed with rich flavors and made with fresh vegetables. Aloo Gobi is a classic Indian vegetarian dish made with potatoes, cauliflower, and a blend of spices and herbs. The name comes from the Hindi words, where 'Aloo' means 'potatoes' and 'Gobi' means 'cauliflower.' This flavorful dish is a beloved everyday meal across the Indian subcontinent, with many variations in its preparation

This dish is a perfect blend of health and flavor! Aloo Gobi isn't just a meal; it's a connection to our heritage, a taste of home, and a reminder of the simple joys and health benefits found in traditional Indian cuisine.

Here are some health benefits that Aloo Gobi offers, making it a great addition to your weight loss diet plan:

nutrient-rich ingredients

Aloo Gobi brings together wholesome potatoes and cauliflower, rich in vitamins, minerals, and antioxidants, making it a nutritious choice for supporting overall health.

fiber for fullness

The high fiber content in both potatoes and cauliflower helps promote fullness, making it easier to manage hunger and potentially reduce calorie intake.

low-calorie option

Naturally low in calories, Aloo Gobi is a satisfying choice for those looking to manage their weight without sacrificing flavor.

metabolism-boosting spices

The spices in this dish, like turmeric and cumin, can help boost metabolism, giving a little extra support to your weight loss journey.

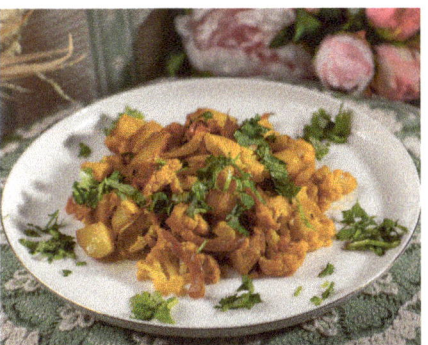

cooking flexibility

Aloo Gobi can be prepared with minimal oil and adjusted to meet specific dietary needs, making it a flexible and nutritious choice for weight loss.

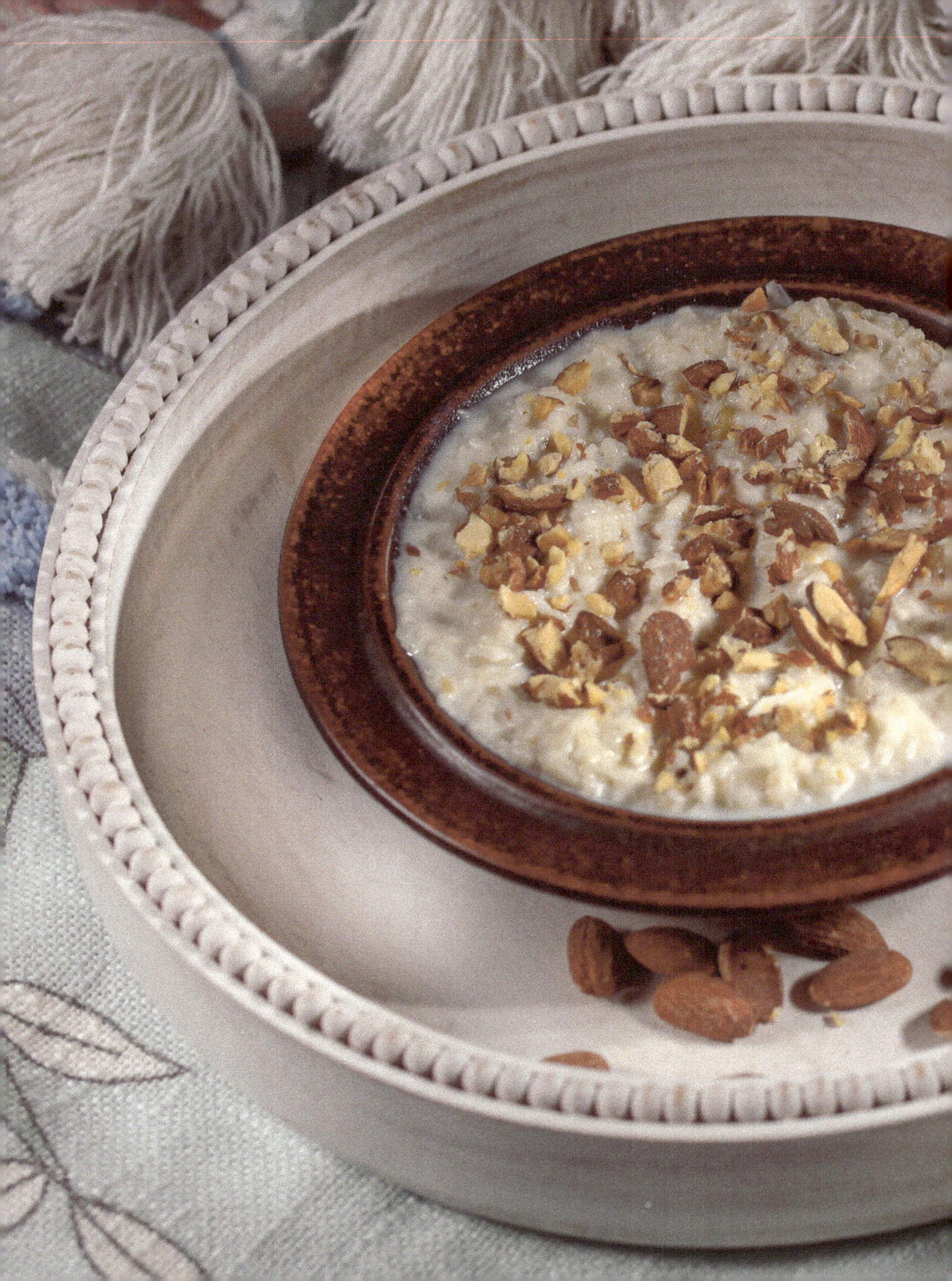

kheerlicious

Every bite is a chance to care for yourself. These recipes are filled with heart, made to support your health, and perfect for sharing with family and friends. Clean eating has never tasted this comforting.

This creamy rice pudding is more than just a dessert—it's a reminder of family celebrations, quiet moments, and how the simplest ingredients can come together to create something extraordinary.

kheerlicious

This classic North Indian dessert is made by gently simmering basmati rice in milk, sweetened with your choice of sweetener, and flavored with cardamom, saffron, and a variety of nuts. The result is a rich, fragrant, and indulgent treat, perfect for festivals and special occasions. This recipe blends carefully selected ingredients to create a velvety, creamy texture that is full of authentic flavors. It's a cherished family recipe that I am excited to share.

ingredients

4 cups *(1 litre)* whole milk
1/4 cup basmati rice
1/4 cup chopped or sliced almonds
1/4 cup golden raisins
1/2 cup shredded coconut flakes
(mixed with 1 tsp cardamom powder)
4-5 tbsp pure maple syrup
1 tsp olive oil
Pinch of cinnamon powder

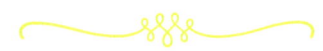

Keep in mind, kheer is usually simmered for a while, so the milk reduces and thickens during the cooking process.

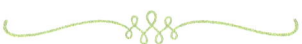

directions

Rinse basmati rice a couple of times in fresh water and then soak in water for 30 minutes. This step allows the rice to absorb moisture, helping it cook evenly and achieve the perfect texture for kheer.

Lightly coat the bottom of a heavy-bottomed pot (preferably stainless steel) with about 2 tablespoons of water to prevent the milk from scalding. Set the heat to medium. Add oil, then add drained rice, and toast for 5 minutes. Next, stir in the coconut flakes and cardamom powder mixture, and toast on low heat for an additional 6-8 minutes.

Add 4 cups of milk to the pan and keep the heat on low to medium. Stir occasionally to prevent the milk from sticking to the bottom of the pan. Allow the milk to come to a gentle boil.

Once the milk starts boiling, stir occasionally for 8-10 minutes. Add the raisins and cook for an additional 5 minutes. Then, stir in the maple syrup and continue stirring frequently for another 5-8 minutes.

Stir in almonds and cook on low to medium heat for 10 minutes, or until the rice becomes tender and the kheer thickens to a creamy consistency.

Serve warm or chilled, as desired.

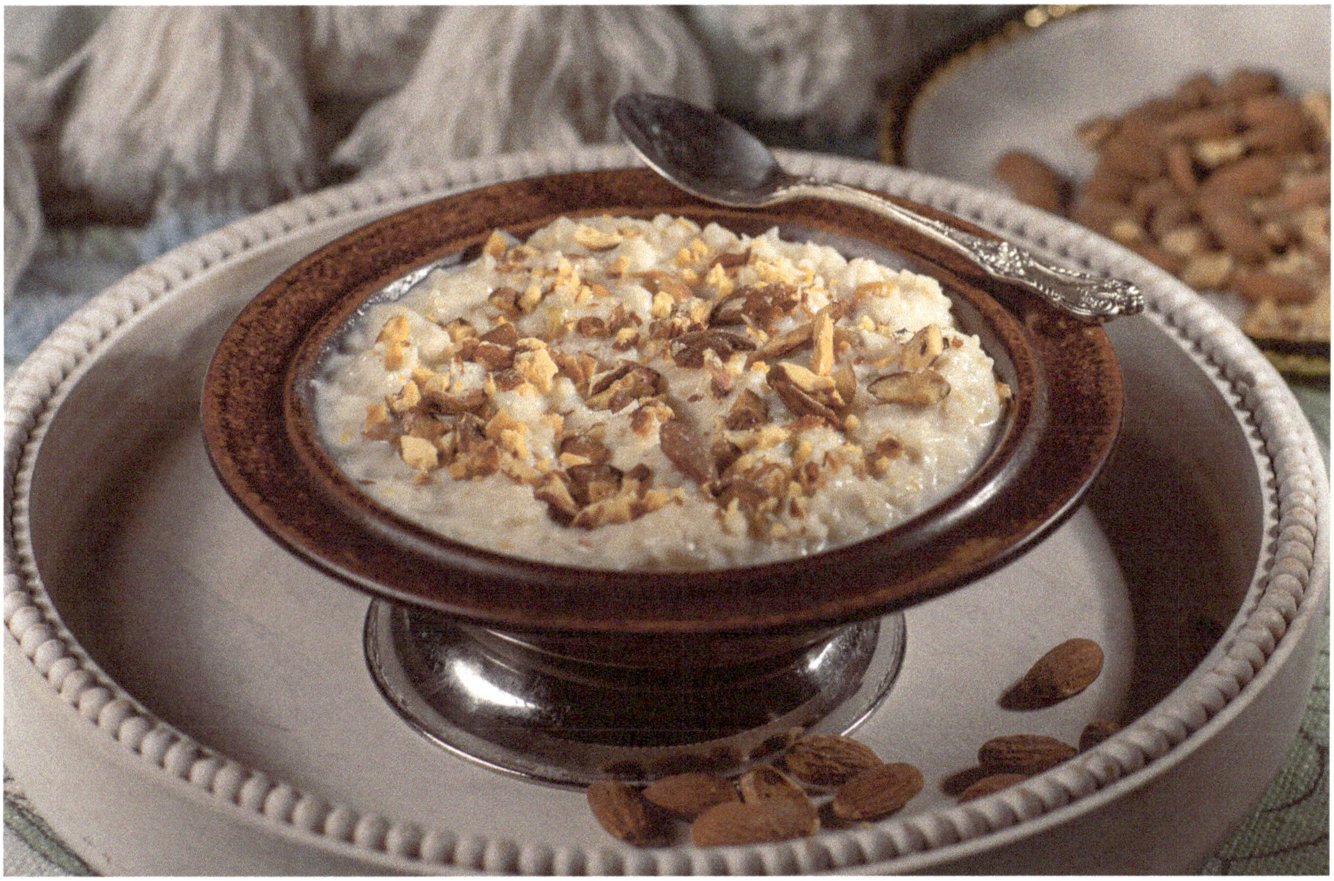

Kheer, often referred to as rice pudding, is a beloved traditional Indian festive dessert with roots in Sanskrit, where the word 'Skheer' means 'milk'—highlighting its key ingredient.

nourishing dessert, heavenly taste!

I love how Kheer can be transformed into a nutritious and wholesome dessert by carefully selecting the right ingredients. Here is why:

rich in nutrients

Milk (or plant-based alternatives) provides **calcium, protein, and vitamin D**, essential for strong bones and muscle health.

Basmati rice isn't just fragrant and delicious, it's also packed with nutrients! Basmati rice has a lower glycemic index compared to other rice varieties, helping regulate blood sugar levels. A great source of vitamins B1 and B6, important for brain function and energy production.

Nuts like almonds and cashews add **healthy fats, protein, and vitamin E**, which are beneficial for brain health and skin.

natural sweetener options

Replacing refined sugar with **maple syrup, honey, or dates** makes kheer a **lower glycemic index** dessert, preventing sugar spikes.

gut-friendly & easy to digest

The **slow-cooked** process of kheer makes it easy on digestion. Spices like **cardamom and cinnamon** not only enhance flavor but also aid digestion and metabolism

high in antioxidants

Cardamom contain antioxidants that help fight inflammation.

Raisins provide natural sweetness, fiber, and iron, improving digestion and blood circulation. Rich in antioxidants, iron, and natural sugars, raisins add a natural sweetness while boosting energy levels.

customizable for dietary needs

It can be made dairy-free with coconut, almond, or oat milk.

A higher-protein version can include quinoa or chia seeds instead of rice.

Adding flaxseeds or walnuts boosts omega-3 fatty acids for heart and brain health.

goodbye to sugar cravings

With natural sweetness from the ingredients, Kheer is a guilt-free treat that satisfies your sweet tooth without compromise.

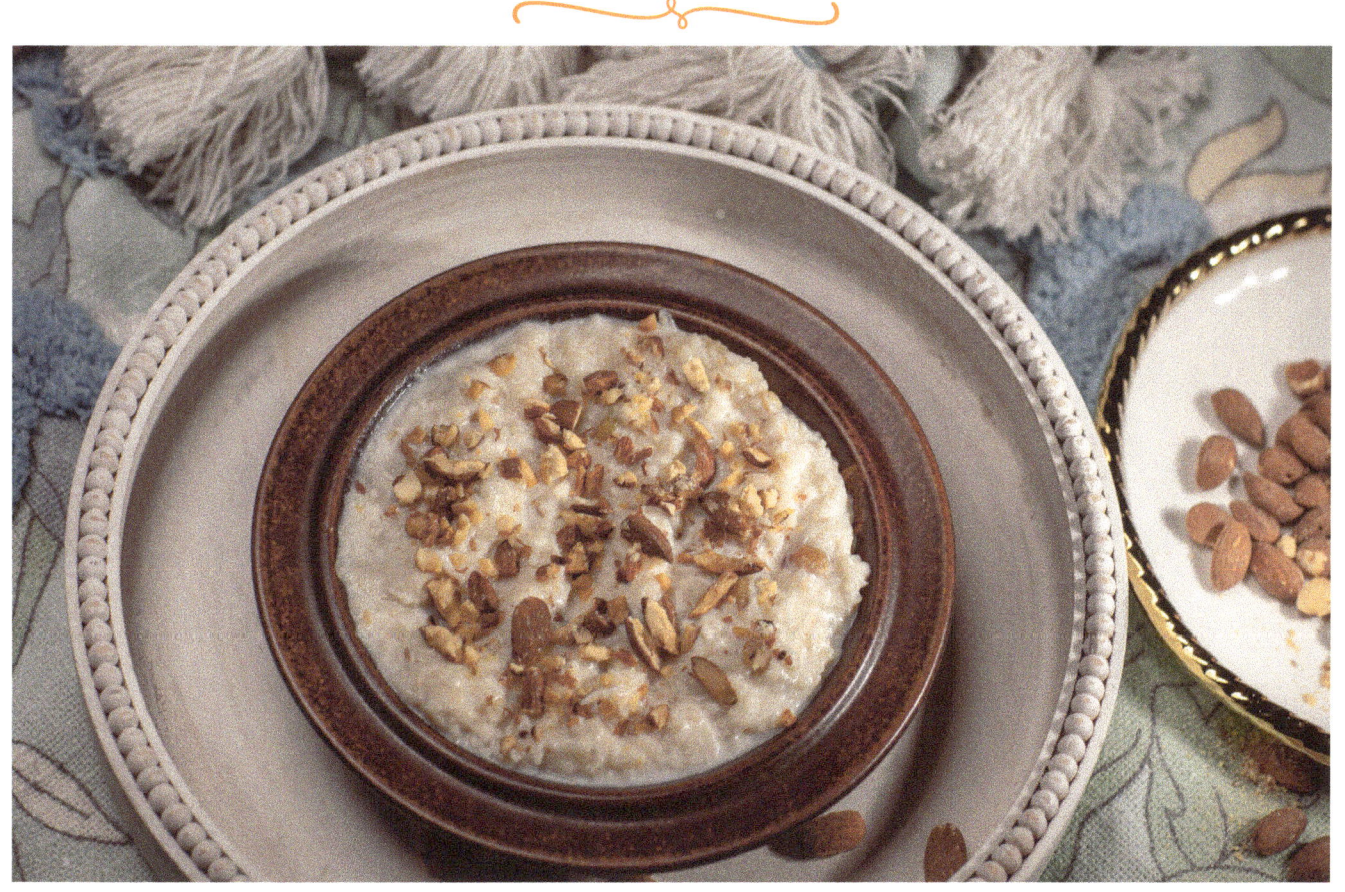

kid-friendly nutrient fueled favorites

- rainbow grilled cheese sandwich   103
- oatfully yours baked donuts   109
- almond glow baked donuts   115
- rainbow smoothies: a colorful adventure in every sip   121
  - berry sunrise smoothie   126
  - mango oat dream smoothie   129
  - oatmazing berry blend smoothie   130
- mini zucchini veggie power pizzas   133
- banana sushi bites   139

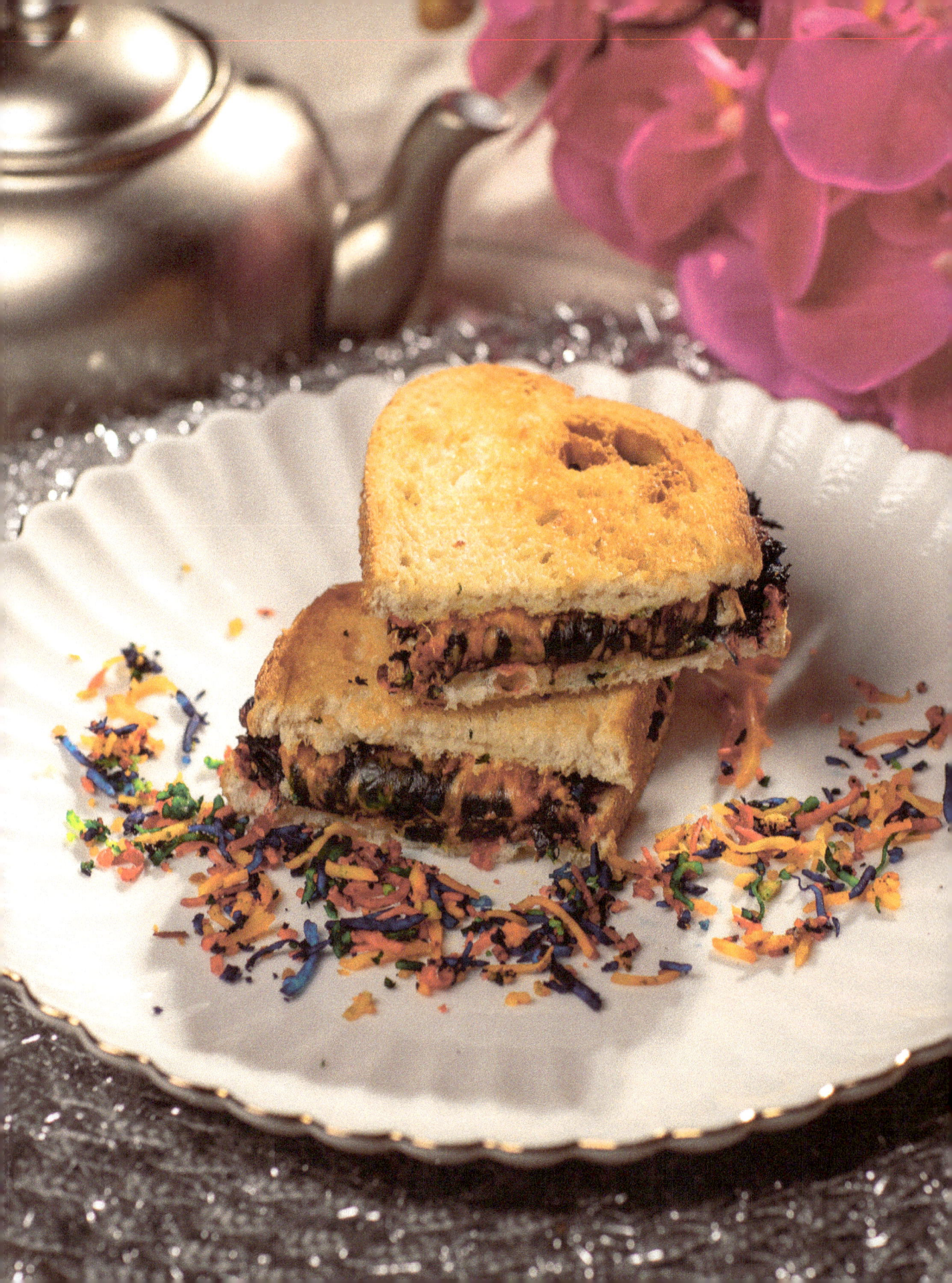

rainbow grilled cheese sandwich

Eating the rainbow isn't just fun—it's smart. Each color brings its own set of nutrients and benefits. These recipes make it easy (and delicious) to fill your plate with color, crunch, and feel-good fuel.

A celebration of colors, crunch, and cheesy comfort. Grilled to perfection, packed with personality.
This sandwich was born on a rainy afternoon, when my little one asked for something colorful and cozy.

With every gooey bite, it's a reminder that food can be both fun and full of love.

rainbow grilled cheese sandwich

Ready to take your grilled cheese to the next level? The rainbow grilled cheese sandwich is a dazzling twist on the classic comfort food—so stunning, it's too pretty to eat! Perfect for both kids and adults, this vibrant creation is as delicious as it is eye-catching. I will guide you step by step to make a rainbow grilled cheese that is both visually spectacular and irresistibly tasty.

ingredients

3 cups grated low-fat mozzarella cheese (or a combination of mozzarella and Swiss cheese)
2 cups fresh baby spinach
1 cup blueberries
4 slices whole wheat bread
3 fresh beets
2 tsp vegan butter, room temperature (or you can use any kind of butter)
1/2 tsp turmeric

directions

Gather the ingredients.

coloring preparation

Beets: Grate beets into a piece of cheesecloth or muslin and squeeze the juice out.

Blueberries: Squeeze fresh or frozen blueberries in cheesecloth or muslin for a light dye, or blend and strain them for a stronger color. Fresh berries produce a softer, bluer shade, while boiling the juice to half its volume creates a deeper, slightly purple hue.

Turmeric: For a traditional dye, dissolve 1 teaspoon of turmeric in cup of water, boil, and reduce by half. Use a small amount for yellow and more for an orange hue.

Spinach: Blend spinach in a blender or food processor, then strain the puree through a fine-mesh sieve and use the juice as a natural dye for cheese.

prepare colored cheese

Divide the shredded cheese into separate bowls (one for each color of the rainbow).

Add a few drops of fresh food coloring to each bowl of cheese and mix with a fork until the cheese is evenly coated in color.

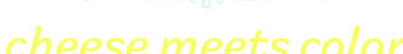

cheese meets color

A cheesy masterpiece that is bursting with flavor and all the colors of the rainbow—bring your lunch to life!

Savor the rainbow, nourish your body! Colored with natural ingredients like beets, blueberries, spinach and turmeric, this grilled cheese is both a visual treat and a healthy delight.

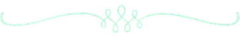

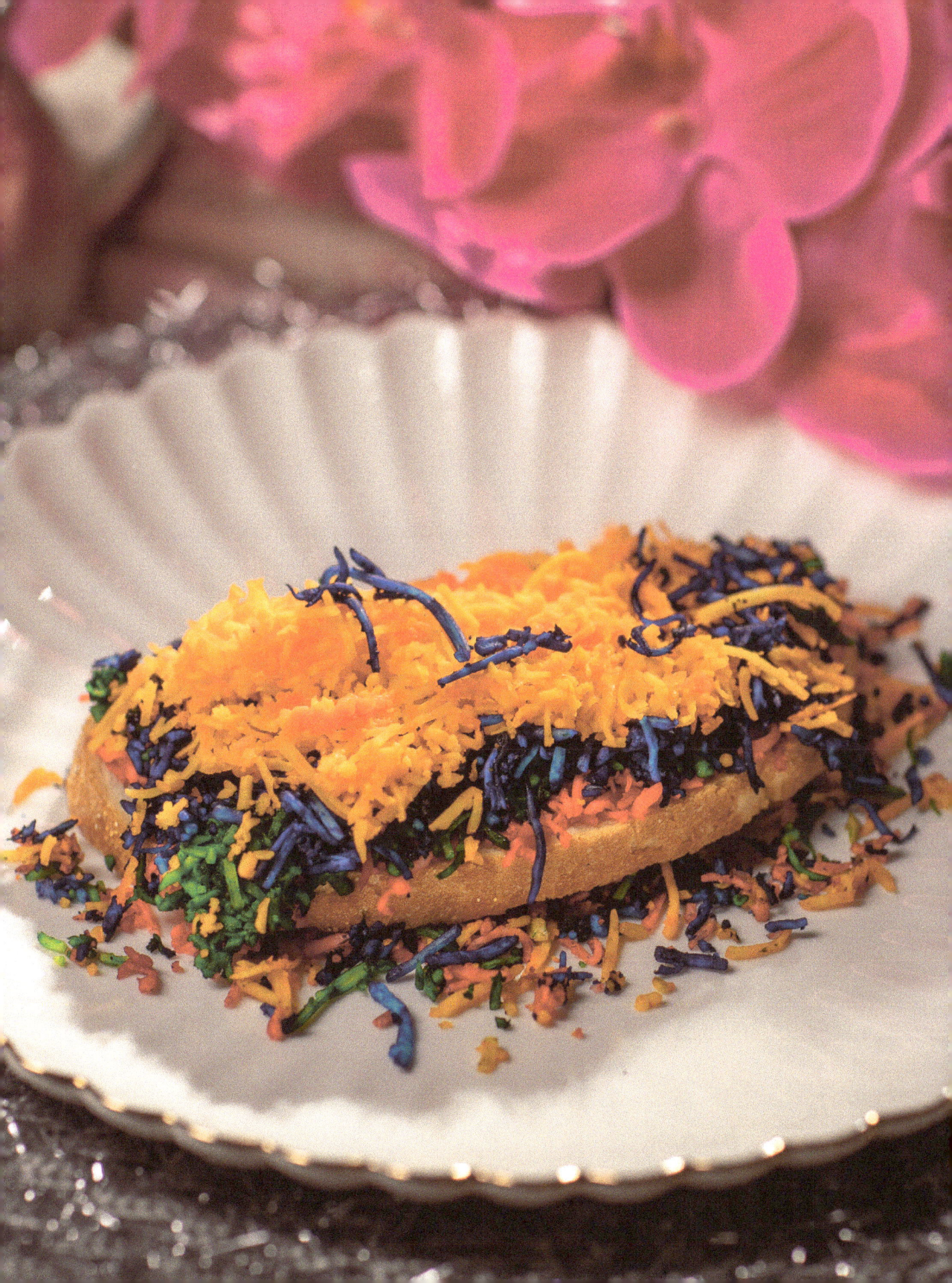

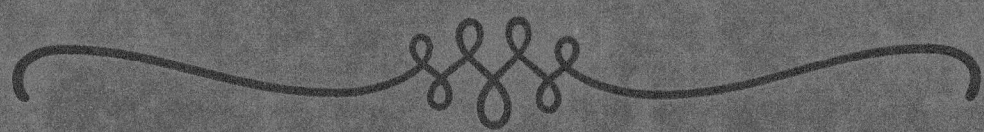

cheese meets color

A cheesy masterpiece that is bursting with flavor and all the colors of the rainbow—bring your lunch to life!

Savor the rainbow, nourish your body! Colored with natural ingredients like beets, blueberries, spinach and turmeric, this grilled cheese is both a visual treat and a healthy delight.

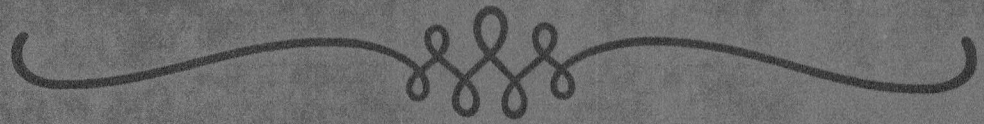

assemble the sandwich

Carefully arrange each colored cheese in lines across one slice of bread, making sure the colors don't overlap. Create a rainbow pattern, using colored cheeses.

grill the sandwich

Heat a medium-sized pan over medium heat and add 1 teaspoon of butter.

Place the slice of bread with the rainbow cheese face down in the pan.

Butter the outer side of the second slice of bread.

Grill for about 3-4 minutes on each side, until the bread is golden brown, and the cheese is melted inside.

serve

Once both sides of the sandwich are golden and crispy, remove from the pan.

Slice along the cheese lines to reveal the rainbow inside.

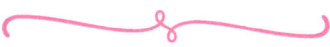

Rainbow Grilled Cheese Sandwich is a healthy recipe made with whole grain bread, low-fat cheese, and natural fruit and vegetable colors to boost its nutritional value.
It offers several benefits:

encourages healthy eating

Using natural fruit and vegetable-based colors introduces kids to nutrient-rich ingredients in a fun way.

boosts creativity

The vibrant colors make mealtime exciting and inspire kids to explore different foods.

provides essential nutrients

Whole grain bread, low-fat cheese, and colorful veggies add fiber, protein, vitamins, and antioxidants.

engages kids in cooking

Letting kids help with food coloring or assembling the sandwich makes them more likely to enjoy and eat it.

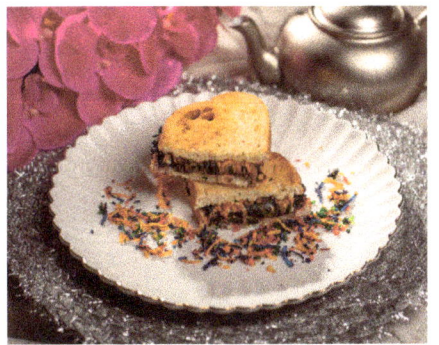

adds a playful element

A visually stunning sandwich turns an ordinary meal into a magical, engaging experience

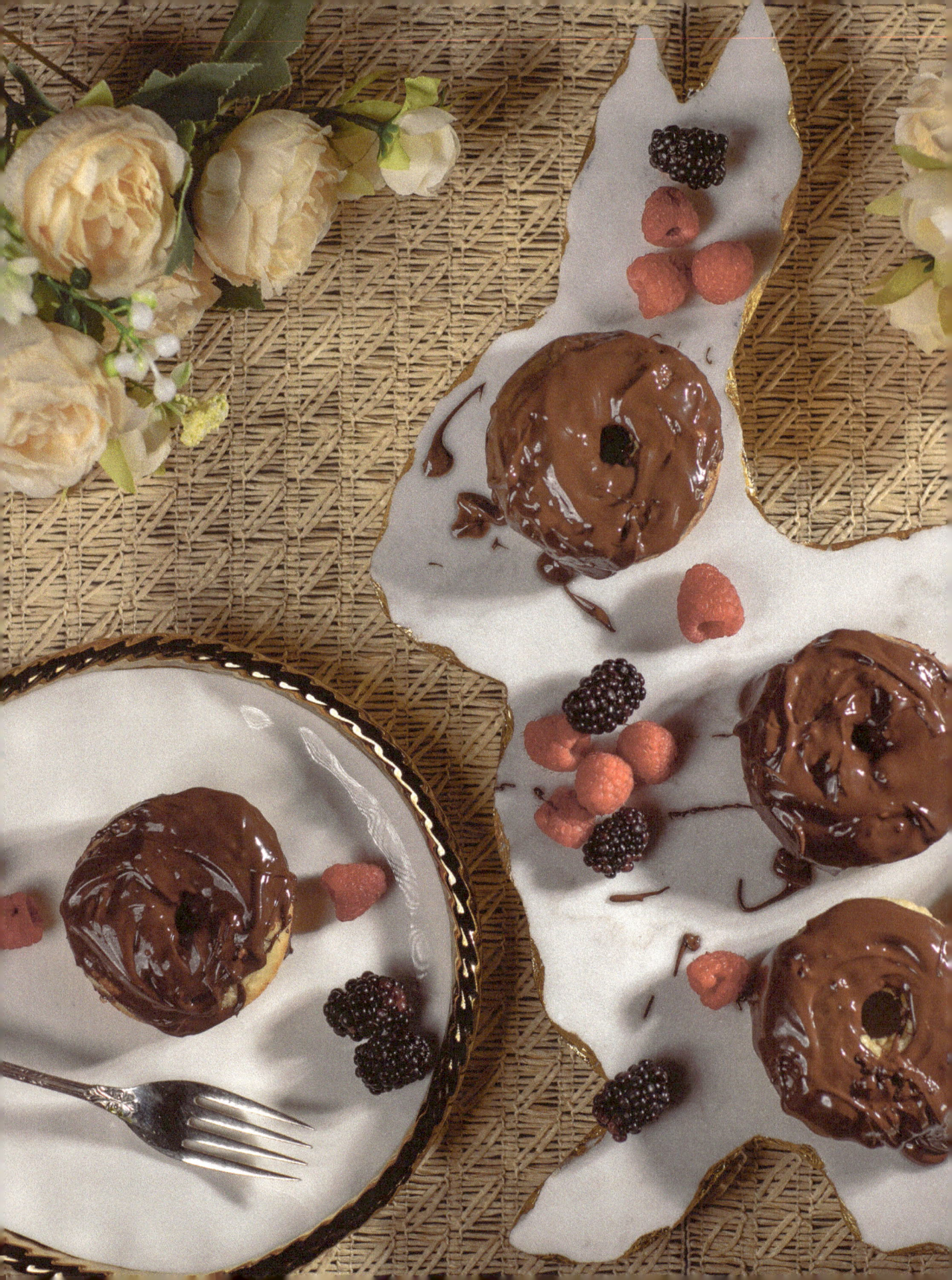

oatfully yours
baked donuts

Some of my favorite memories are of little hands helping in the kitchen, peeking over the counter, giggling while mixing, and sneaking bites when they think I'm not looking. That's the magic of cooking with kids—it turns mealtime into a moment of connection and learning.

Cozy, soft and naturally sweetened.
You know that moment when your kid asks for a second donut, and you say yes... without hesitation? That's the magic of these little guys.

oatfully yours baked donuts

Craving a fun, healthy, and delicious way to kickstart your day? These baked oatmeal donuts are simple to prepare and loaded with nutritious ingredients. Who says donuts can't be healthy? Baked donuts are the perfect answer! Baked and filled with feel-good goodness! These donuts are proof that healthy eating can still be full of fun and flavor.

ingredients

2 cups oat flour
2 eggs
1/2 cup maple syrup
1/4 cup almond milk (unsweetened)
1 tsp baking powder
1 tsp vanilla extract
Any cooking spray
Silicon donut pan

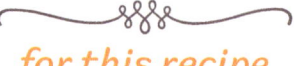

for this recipe

If you want to make your own oat flour, it is super easy to make! Simply blend oats in a high-speed blender until they turn into a fine powder, then store in an airtight container until ready to use.

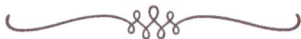

directions

Preheat oven to 350° F. Spray donut pans with cooking spray.

In a large bowl, combine the oat flour and baking powder.

Add the wet ingredients into the dry ingredients and gently mix until just combined. Gently fold until you get a smooth and shiny batter. Don't over-mix the batter, or your donuts won't be as fluffy.

Grease the donut pan. Transfer the batter into a Ziploc bag, snip a small corner of the bag and pipe the batter into the donut tray, filling each mold to the top for thick, fluffy donuts. Be careful not to overfill the molds to maintain the classic donut shape.

Bake for 12-15 minutes at 350°F (180°C), or until a toothpick inserted in the center comes out clean.

Remove the donut pan from the oven and place it on a cooling rack. Allow the donuts to cool completely before removing them from the mold to prevent them from breaking.

Note: If you are not piping the batter, just use a spoon to fill the cavity.

Dip the donuts into the glaze (recipe on the next page) and place them back on the wire rack to set. Enjoy!

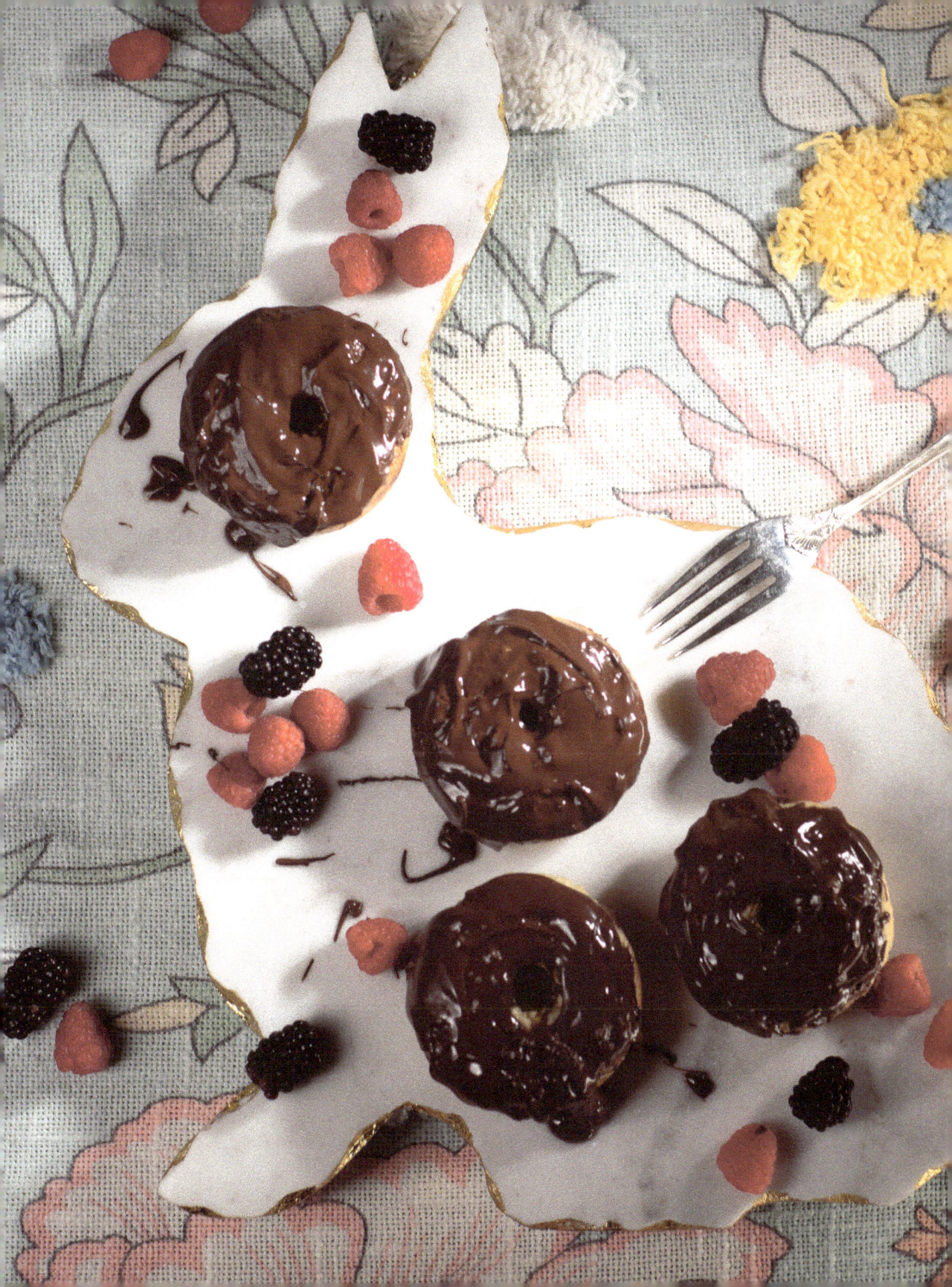

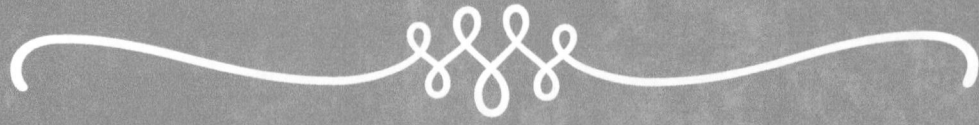

for this recipe

If you want to make your own oat flour, it is super easy to make! Simply blend oats in a high-speed blender until they turn into a fine powder, then store in an airtight container until ready to use.

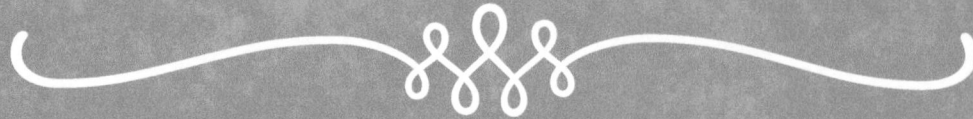

Baking with oat flour is incredibly easy. While traditional donut recipes use wheat flour, oat flour offers a nutritious and gluten-free alternative. It helps keep kids full since oats are rich in fiber.

reasons to love
this baked donut recipe

Perfect for both kids and adults to enjoy.

Quick & Easy
Simple ingredients, minimal prep, and ready in no time!

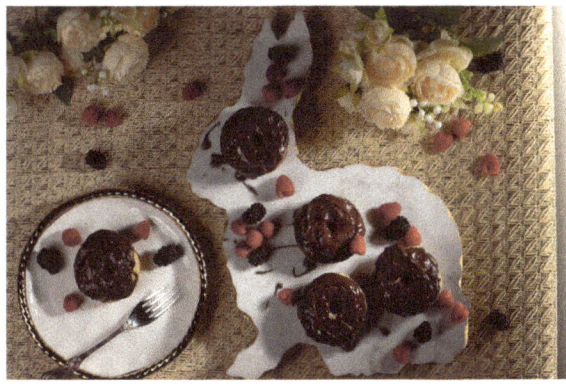

Nutritious & Wholesome
Made with oat flour, giving them a wonderfully soft and fluffy texture.

Kid-Friendly & Fun
A fun and delicious weekend indulgence.

Lighter and healthier than traditional fried donuts.

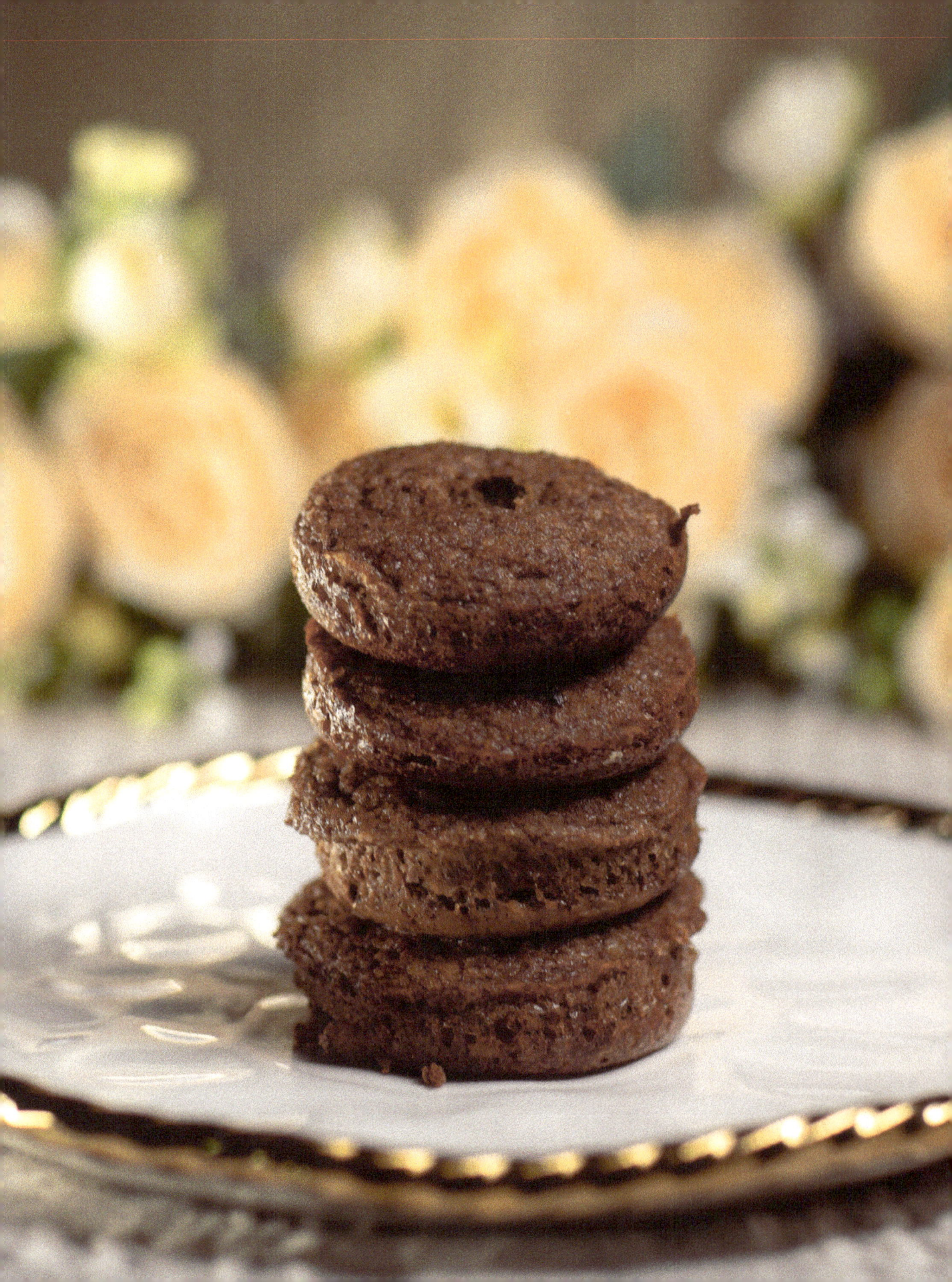

almond glow baked donuts

These donuts were born out of a craving and a little mom-hack magic—sweet enough to feel like a treat but nourishing enough to feel proud of

Grab one for breakfast, pack one for lunch, or surprise them after school. These donuts are my sweet way of saying 'I love you'—the healthy way.
These donuts may look like dessert, but they're secretly packed with nourishing ingredients—perfect for little tummies and big smiles!

almond glow baked donuts

These gluten-free, low-carb, high-protein donuts make for a super healthy snack when you are in the mood for something sweet! They taste amazing, especially when topped with melted chocolate. You can customize them with a drizzle of dark chocolate and garnish with toasted coconut, chopped almonds, or dark chocolate chips, depending on your preferences. Enjoy!

ingredients

for almond donuts
2 cups almond flour
2 eggs
1/4 cup maple syrup
2 tbsp cocoa powder
1 tsp vanilla extract
1 tsp baking powder
Olive oil cooking spray
Silicon donut pan

for chocolate glaze
1/4 cup semi-sweet or dark chocolate chips
1/4 cup olive oil

Almonds are packed with antioxidants, healthy fats, and protein, turning these donuts into a satisfying and wholesome snack that helps fuel your day!

directions

for almond donuts

Preheat the oven to 375°F (190°C). Generously spray or brush a nonstick/silicon donut pan with cooking spray and set it aside.

In a mixing bowl, whisk the eggs, maple syrup and vanilla extract until the mixture is light and slightly foamy, about 3-4 minutes. Add the almond flour, baking powder, and cocoa powder, and mix everything together thoroughly with a spatula until the batter becomes very thick and all the almond flour is incorporated.

Transfer the batter into a plastic Ziploc bag and cut off one of the corners. Pipe the batter evenly into the prepared donut pan.

Bake in the center of the preheated oven for 12-15 minutes, or until a toothpick inserted the center comes out clean. Remove the donut pan from the oven and place it on a cooling rack. Allow the donuts to cool completely before removing them from the mold to prevent them from breaking.

to glaze de donuts

Take a small pan and bring 1 cup of water to a boil. Once the water boils, place a bowl or coffee cup filled with chocolate chips and olive oil in the center of the pan. Melt the chocolate

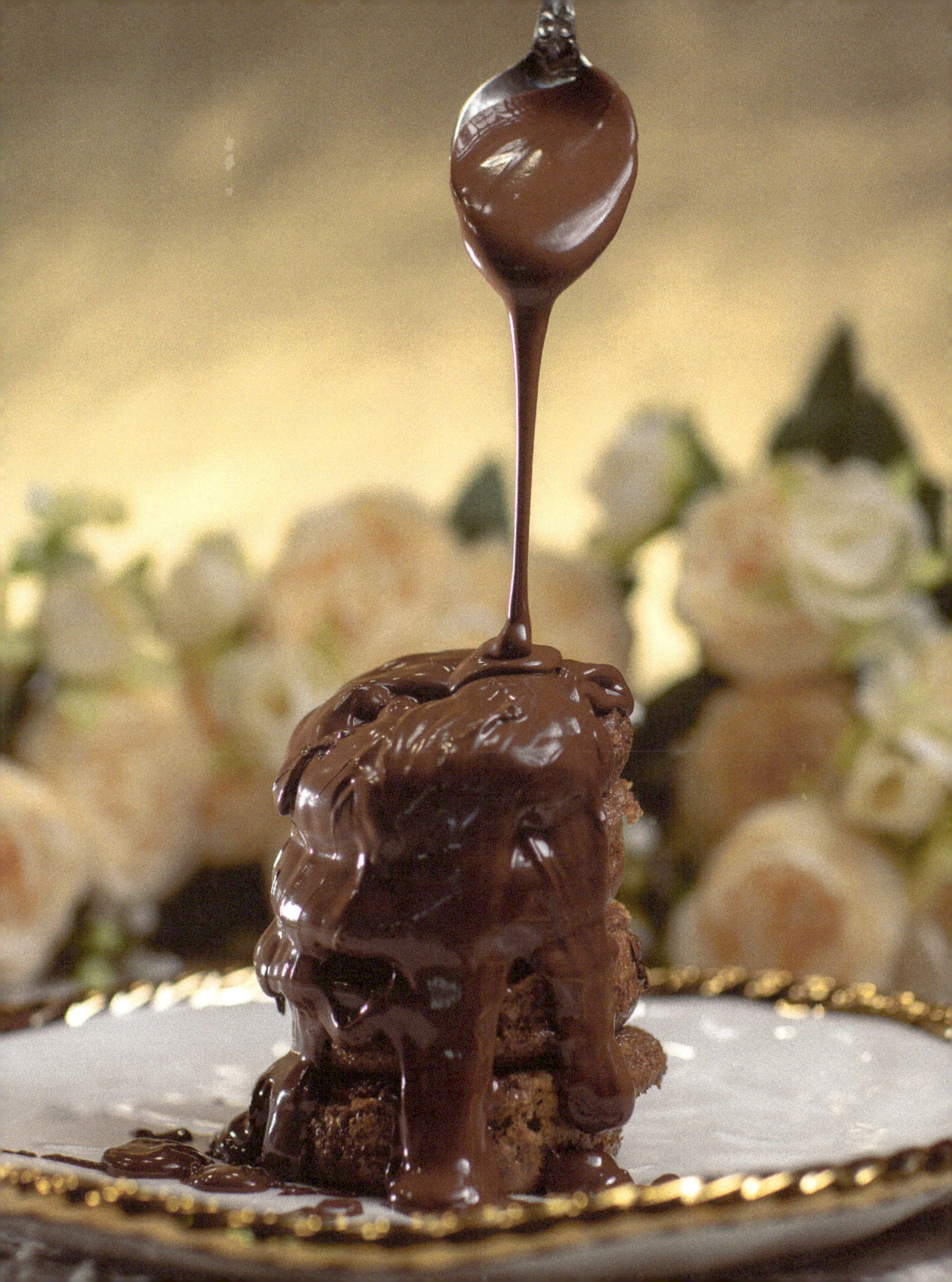

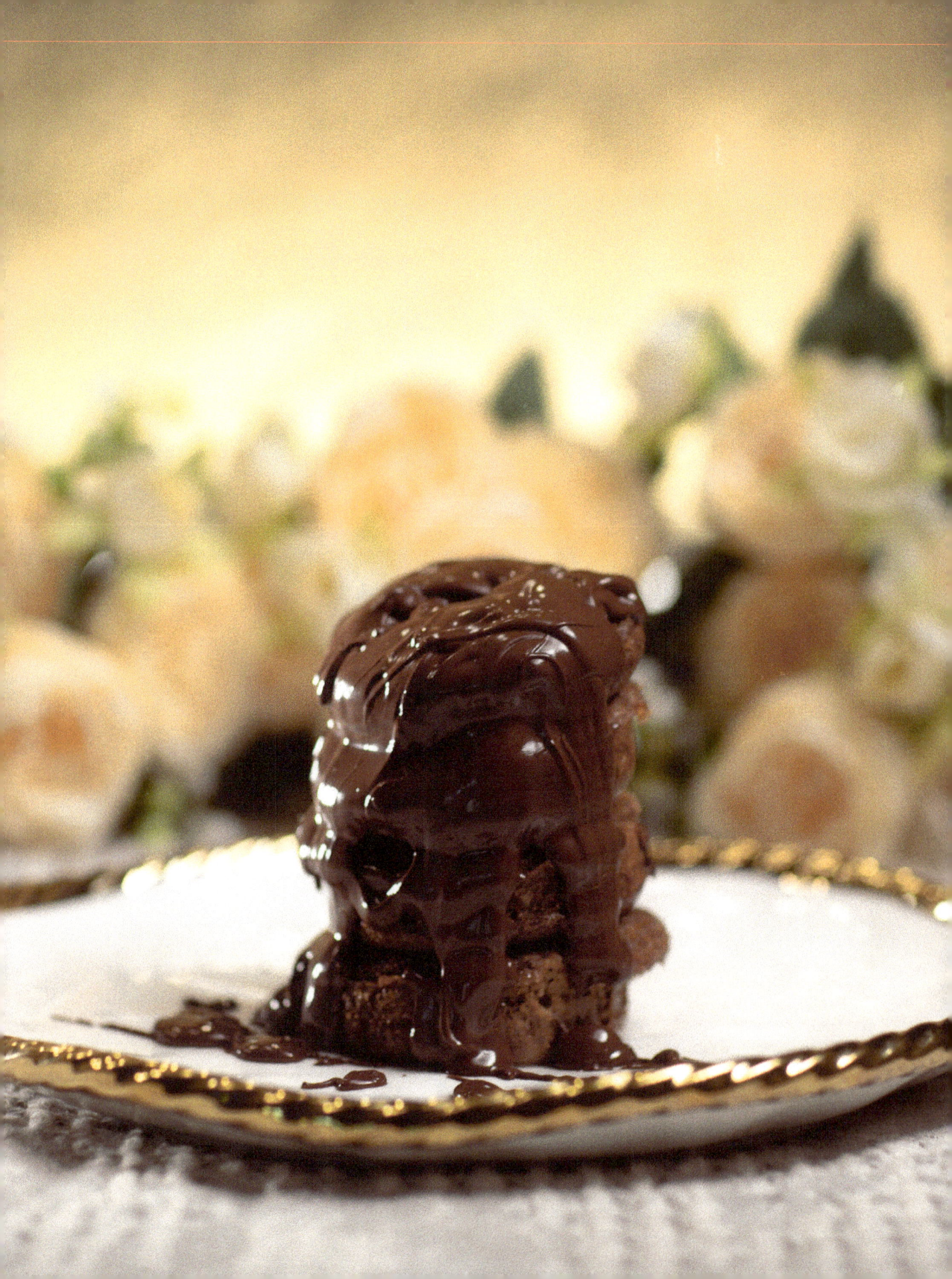

over low heat, stirring continuously to avoid burning. Once smooth, remove from heat.

Dip each donut into the chocolate mixture, allowing any excess to drip off, then transfer them to parchment paper. Repeat this for all donuts. When dipping, be gentle, as the donuts might still be warm inside and delicate. For a more classic look, dip the bottom side (the part that was in the tray), as it's flatter. Alternatively, you can spoon the melted chocolate onto the donuts for a smoother, more even coating.

Enjoy your perfectly coated chocolate donuts!

how to store

I recommend storing your donuts in an airtight container in the fridge for up to 3-4 days. For longer storage, you can freeze them for up to 2 months. When you are ready to enjoy, just thaw them in the fridge and they are good to go.

I can't emphasize enough how beneficial oatmeal is for kids. Oat flour is a versatile, wholesome ingredient that offers multiple health benefits, particularly for heart health, blood sugar regulation, weight management, and digestion. Packed with fiber, vitamins, and minerals, oatmeal supports overall well-being. Its high fiber content promotes healthy digestion and helps prevent constipation. Oatmeal provides a steady energy release, keeping kids fueled and focused throughout the day. Plus, the fiber and protein help kids feel satisfied longer, preventing mid-morning hunger. Oats are also rich in vitamin B, crucial for brain development and cognitive function.

Here are some reasons kids should eat almond baked donuts:

Packed with plant-based protein, almonds help build muscle and support a strong, healthy body. Almonds contain heart-healthy fats that help support brain function and energy levels. Baked almond donuts are a healthier alternative to sugary store-bought donuts, helping to maintain energy without blood sugar spikes. Almonds are high in fiber, which supports healthy digestion and keeps kids feeling full longer.

These healthy donuts offer a delicious and nutritious treat that kids will love!

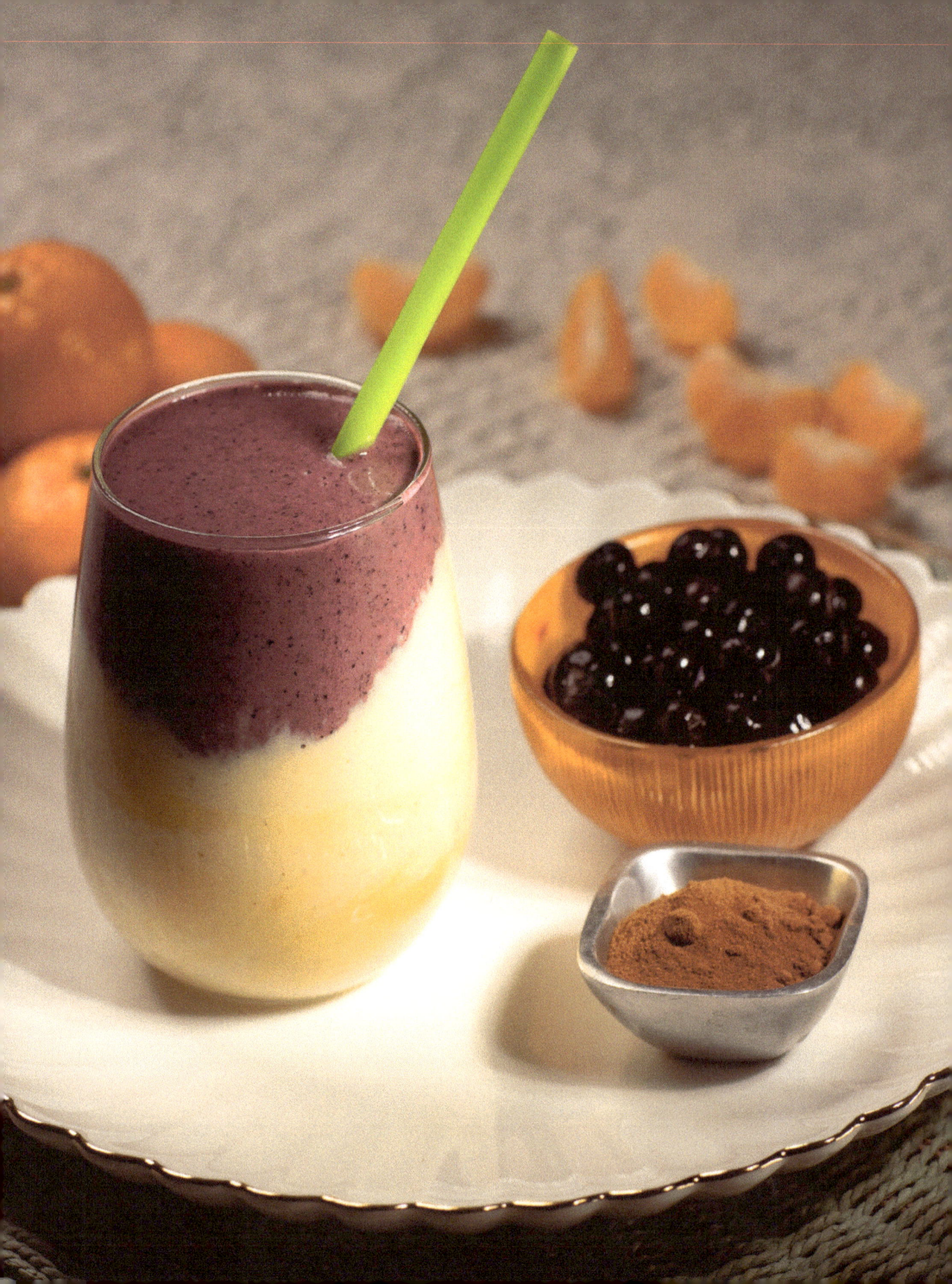

rainbow smoothies
a colorful adventure in every sip

I remember the first time I made a smoothie for them, packed with fruits, veggies, and wholesome ingredients – their faces lit up with delight, and it was a reminder that healthy eating doesn't have to be boring.

Smoothies for kids are like liquid sunshine—bright, fun, and packed with goodness! Our family smoothie time quickly became a fun tradition, where each blend became a new adventure in flavor and nutrition. From hidden greens to antioxidant-packed fruits, we discovered that fueling our bodies with whole ingredients could be both delicious and exciting!

rainbow smoothies
a colorful adventure in every sip

Smoothies are an excellent way to enjoy a nutrient-packed meal or snack, blending vitamin-rich fruits and vegetables, protein, and healthy fats into a drinkable form. They are quick, easy, and affordable to make at home, allowing endless flavor combinations with ingredients you already have. While store-bought smoothies often contain more added sugar than desired, making them yourself gives you full control over the sweetness.

I wanted to share some fun and healthy smoothie recipes for kids that will keep them energized and full, all while using the wholesome, natural ingredients that the earth produces.

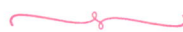

here are some tips on how to make flavorful smoothies:

Start with a liquid base. Great low-calorie, low-sugar options include water, juice, non-dairy milk, regular milk, green tea, or coconut water.

Boost with protein and healthy fats. Nut butter, garbanzo beans, yogurt, silken tofu, and avocado provide creaminess, essential nutrients, and long-lasting energy.

Load up on vegetables. Kale, spinach, parsley, beet greens, cucumber, and celery bring fresh flavors and extra nutrients. Try incorporating them into veggie or green smoothies for added benefits.

Add fresh or frozen fruit. Almost any fruit works well! If using fresh fruit, blend in ice cubes for a smoother, more refreshing texture.

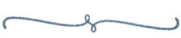

some tips on freezing fresh fruits:

Freezing Bananas: Peel and slice bananas into 1-inch pieces. Arrange them on a baking sheet in a single layer and freeze to prevent sticking. Once frozen, transfer them to a resealable freezer bag for easy storage.

Freezing Fresh Berries: Spread berries out on a baking sheet and freeze until firm. Then, transfer them to a resealable freezer bag to keep them fresh and ready for smoothies.

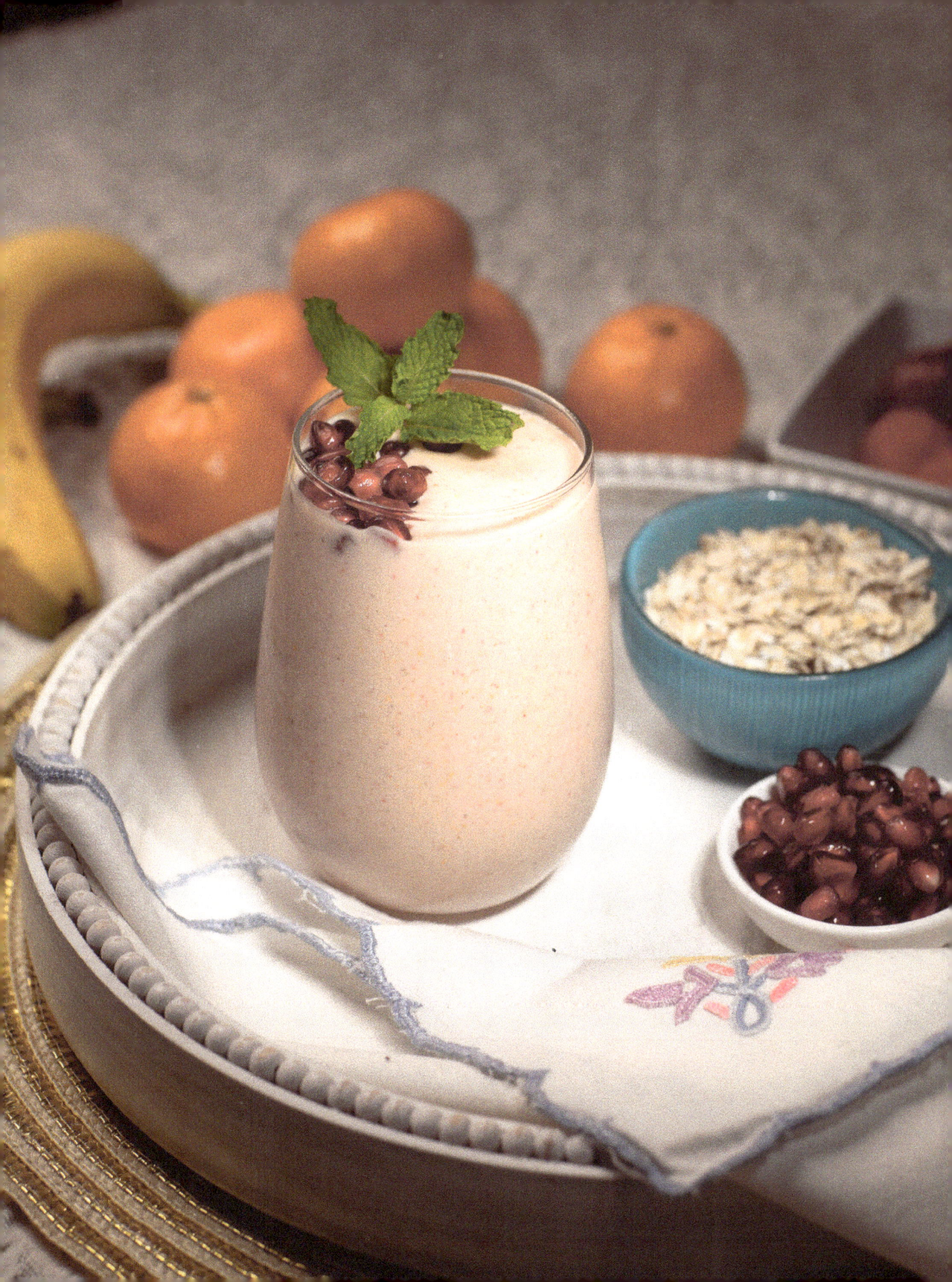

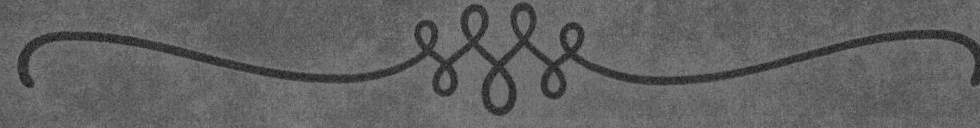

smoothie science

Layering fruits by color helps preserve the vitamins and antioxidants—keep your smoothie full of fresh energy and flavor!

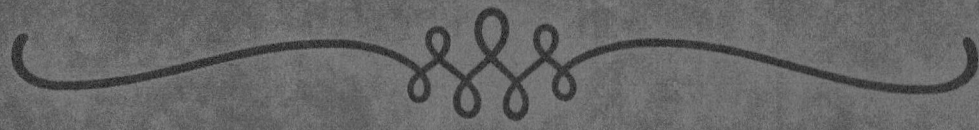

the formula for a healthy smoothie

Add 1/2 cup to 1 cup **liquid**, 1 tbsp to 1/4 cup of a **creamy add-in**, 1/2 tsp to 1 tbsp of a **flavor boost**, 1 to 2 cups of **frozen fruits and vegetables**, and a touch of **sweetener**, if desired.

liquid

Juice
Iced coffee
Milk
Plant-based milk
Water

creamy add-in

Nut butter
Yogurt
Coconut cream
Avocado

flavor boost

Vanilla extract
Lemon juice
Cocoa powder
Ground cardamom
Ground cinnamon
Lime juice
Ginger
Turmeric
Fresh mint

frozen fruits & vegetables

Spinach
Kale
Cauliflower
Banana
Peach
Berries
Cherries
Pineapple
Mango
Kiwi
Apple
Melon

sweetener

Agave
Honey

oatmazing berry blend smoothie

Try this smoothie for breakfast before school; it will keep you full all morning! Plus, you can make it the night before, and it will still be fresh the next day. While you can skip the chia seeds, they pack in loads of nutrients and are the secret ingredient that really keeps you satisfied.

ingredients

3/4 cup oat milk
1/2 cup frozen strawberries
1/2 cup fresh banana slices
1/4 cup uncooked oats (yup, as in oatmeal!)
1/4 cup mandarin oranges (fresh)
1/4 cup Greek yogurt
1 tsp walnuts
1 tsp chia seeds

directions

Add oats and chia seeds to the blender, then blend on high until the mixture reaches the texture of flour. Pour in the milk and use a spoon to stir in the oats and chia mixture from the bottom. Next, add the yogurt, followed by the strawberries, oranges, bananas, and walnuts. Blend on high until smooth and ready to enjoy! Just pour it into a fun cup, toss in a colorful straw, and enjoy every sip!

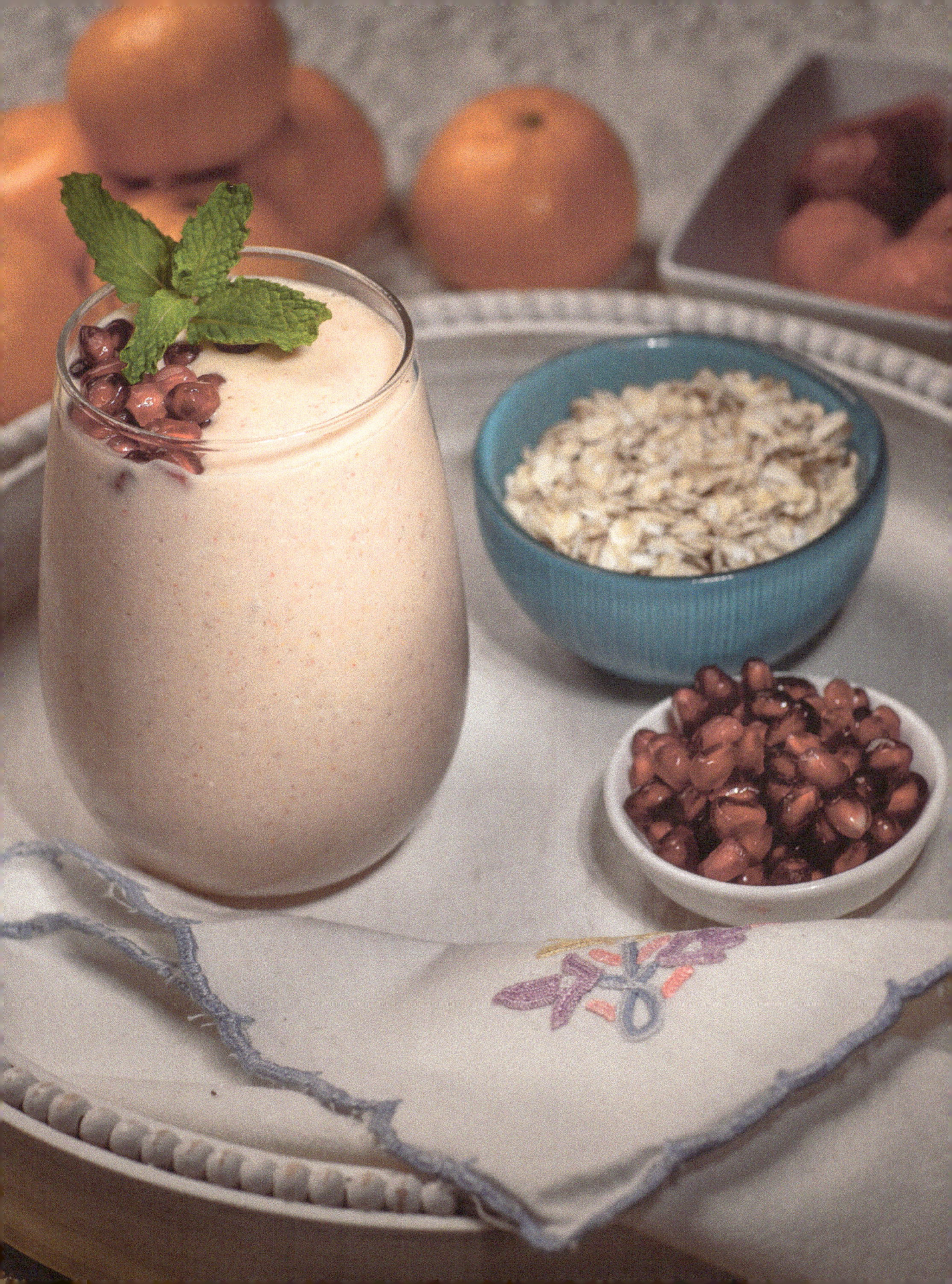

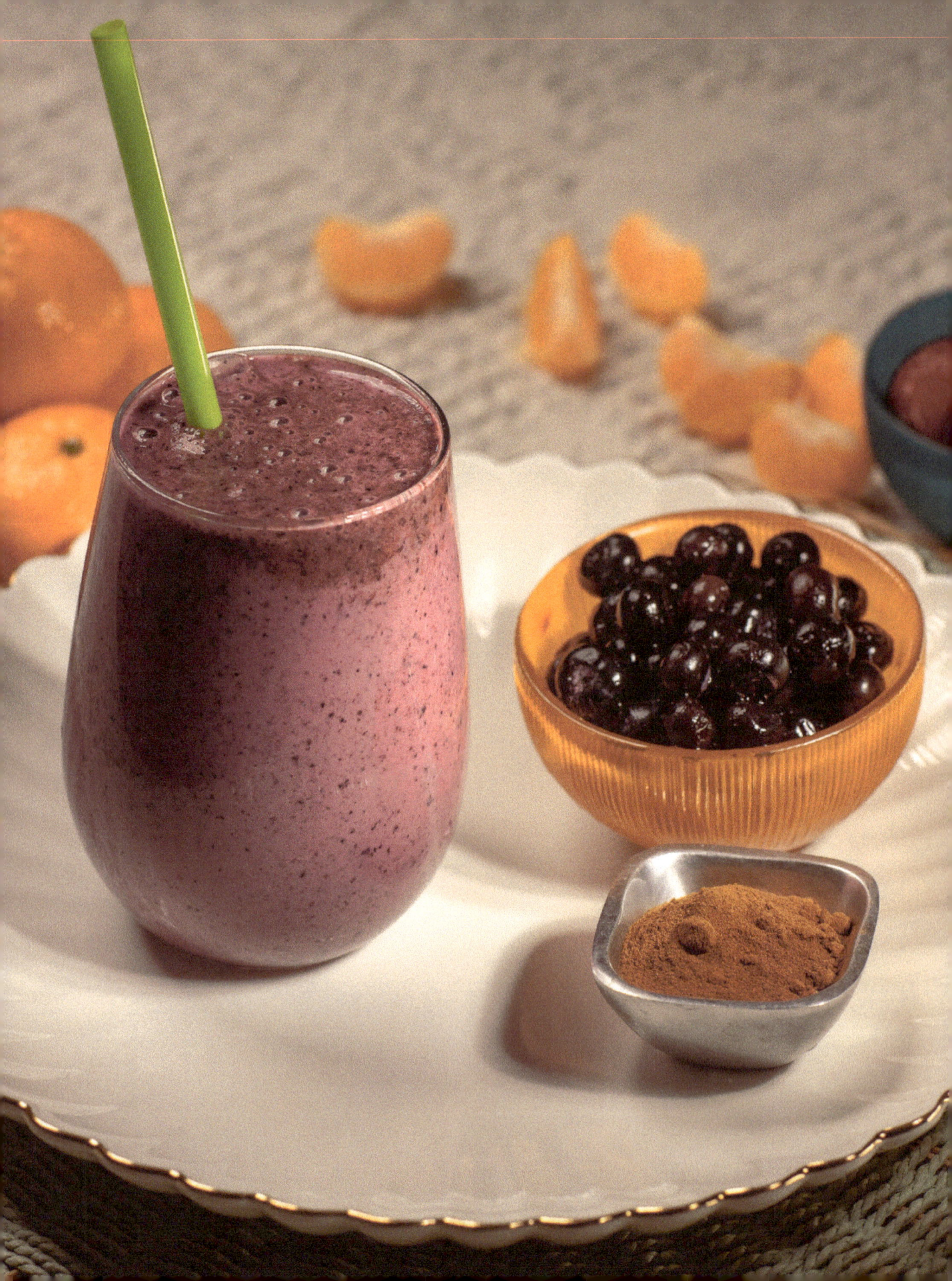

berry sunrise smoothie

ingredients

1 cup Frozen Strawberries and Blueberries- I prefer using frozen ingredients, as they make my smoothie thick and creamy, creating that perfect, satisfying texture.

1/2 cup Oat Milk- For a smooth and well-blended smoothie, a liquid base is essential. I love using oat milk for its mildly nutty flavor and creamy texture, but you can use any milk you prefer or have on hand.

1/2 cup Vanilla Greek Yogurt- Nonfat vanilla Greek yogurt not only adds a boost of protein to the smoothie, making it more filling, but its sweet vanilla flavor pairs perfectly with berries, creating a deliciously creamy blend.

A pinch of Cinnamon- My secret smoothie ingredient—especially for blueberry smoothies! Its subtle warmth gives the smoothie a unique twist, making it stand out among the usual blueberry and strawberry blends you might have tried.

directions

Add all the ingredients to the blender. Blend until smooth. Toss it in a glass, add a straw, and let the smoothie magic begin.

mango oat dream smoothie

ingredients

1 cup frozen mangoes
1 banana
1/2 cup vanilla Greek yogurt
1/2 cup oat milk
1 tsp walnuts

directions

Combine mangoes, banana, vanilla yogurt, and milk in a blender, and blend until smooth.

Pour into a fun cup, add a colorful straw, and enjoy!

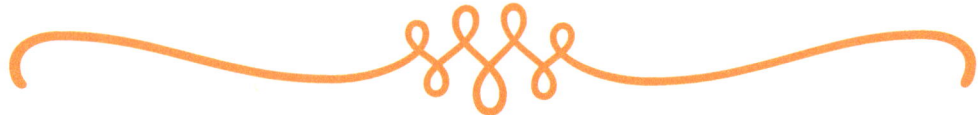

Cool blends to energize your day—colorful, creamy, and packed with nutrients. These smoothies are like a hug in a glass—colorful, cool, and packed with goodness.

Whirl them up for a burst of fruity fun that even picky eaters will love.

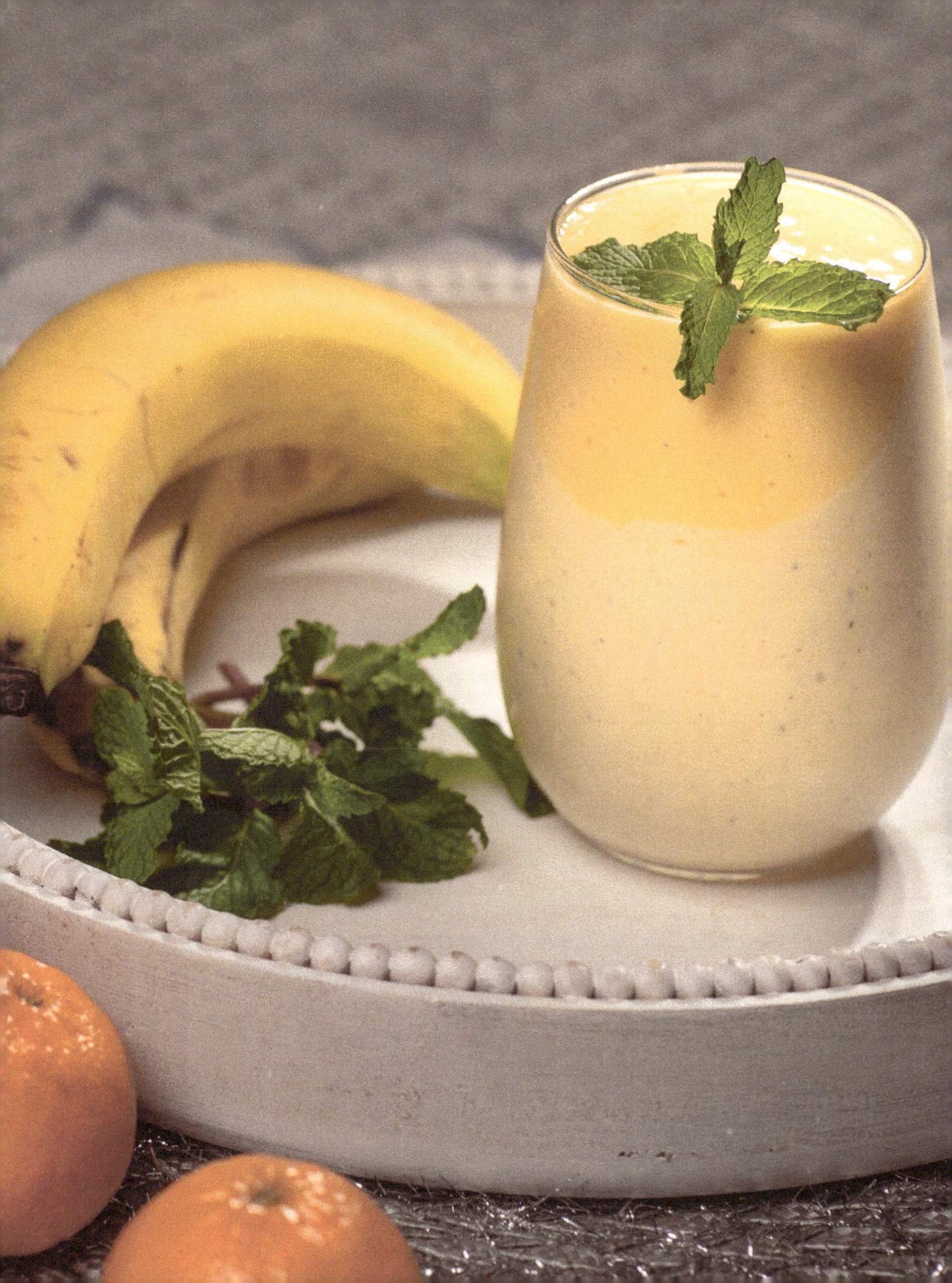

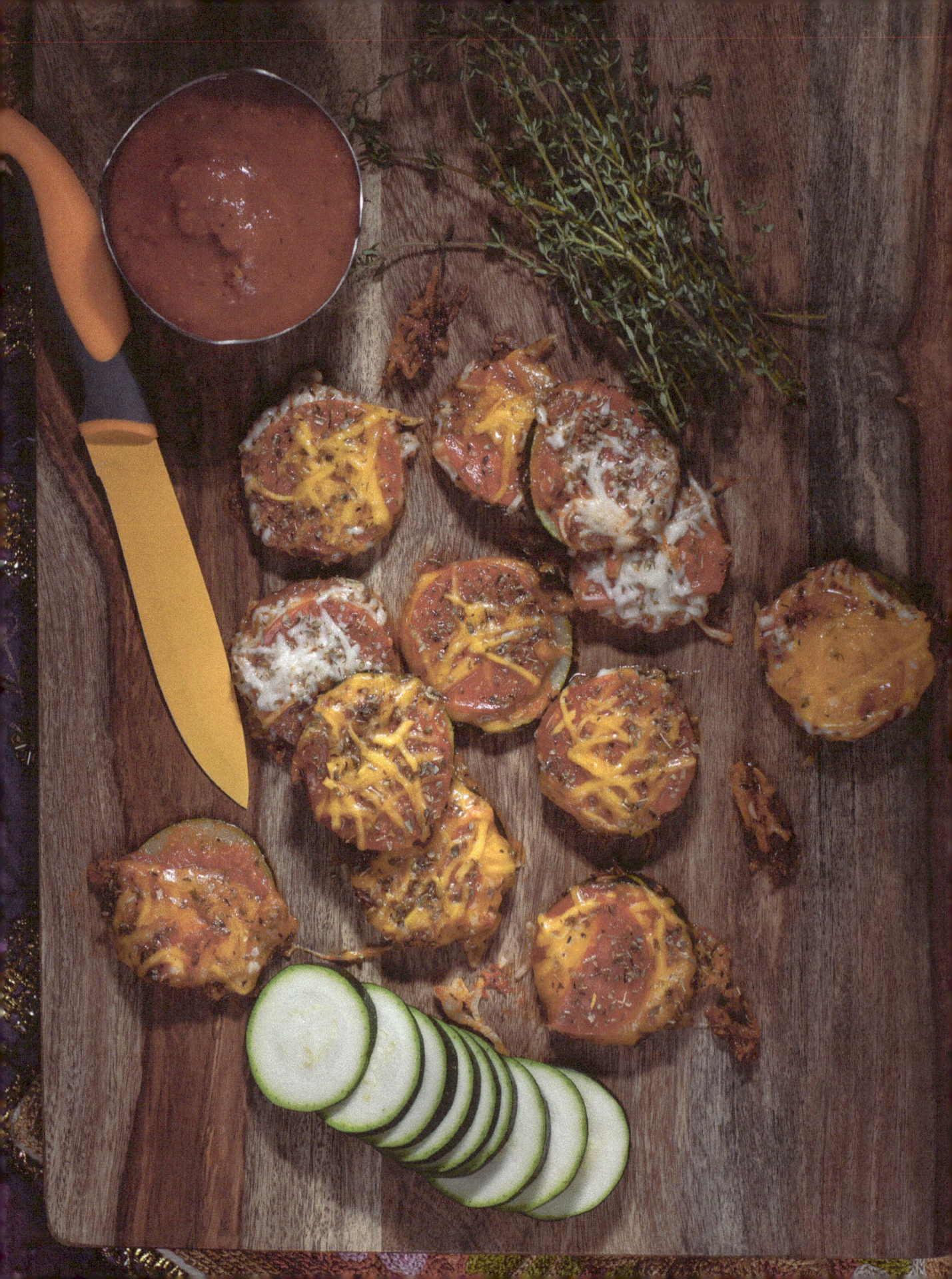

mini zucchini veggie power pizzas

Creating healthy meals for kids is something that's close to my heart. As a mom, I've always wanted to nourish my children with food that not only tastes delicious but also fuels their growing bodies.

Feeding kids nutritious food doesn't have to be a battle—it can be an adventure. It's about offering options that help kids develop a love for food that nourishes them, setting the foundation for a lifetime of good eating habits. And just like that, what starts as a small change becomes part of their everyday routine—a nourishing habit that will help them thrive as they grow.

mini zucchini veggie power pizzas

Zucchini in a pizza? Yes, please! These bite-sized wonders bring a crispy-cheesy joy that even the pickiest eaters can't resist.

Kid-approved, veggie-forward, and fun to assemble! Bite-sized, crispy, and crave-worthy! This recipe was my fun little experiment to get more greens onto the plate—and it worked like magic. Now it's a family favorite that's equally nourishing and delicious.

ingredients

- 2 medium zucchinis, sliced (1/4 inch thick slices)
- 6 pieces turkey pepperonis, cut in half
- 3/4 cup reduced-fat mozzarella cheese, shredded
- 3/4 cup reduced-fat cheddar cheese, shredded
- 1/2 cup no sugar added marinara or pizza sauce
- 1/4 tsp dried basil or parsley leaves
- Olive oil cooking spray

directions

Preheat the oven or air fryer to 400°F on the bake setting. Line a baking sheet with foil, spray it lightly with olive oil cooking spray, and set aside.

Slice the zucchini into -inch thick rounds and arrange them in a single layer on the prepared baking sheet. Lightly spray the zucchinis with cooking oil to help them crisp up.

Bake for 4-5 minutes per side until lightly golden. Remove from the oven or air fryer and let them cool.

Top the zucchini slices with a small spoonful of marinara or pizza sauce, cheese, pepperoni slices and dried herbs.

Bake again for 5-8 minutes, or until the zucchini is crispy and cheese is bubbly and melted.

This recipe makes 14 mini zucchini pizza bites

nutrition nugget
Mini Bites, Major Wins: Perfect for after-school snacks, movie nights, or anytime munching.

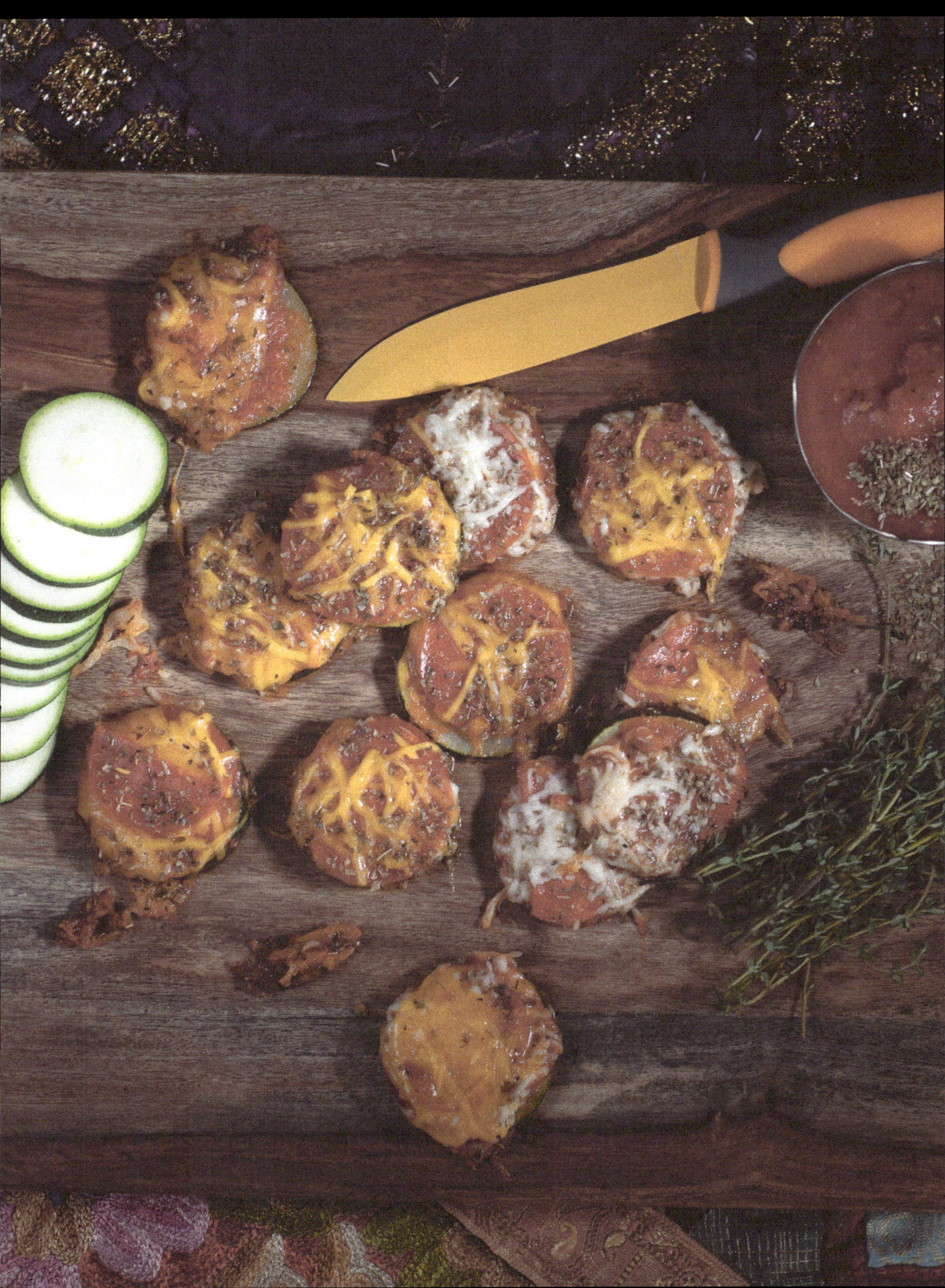

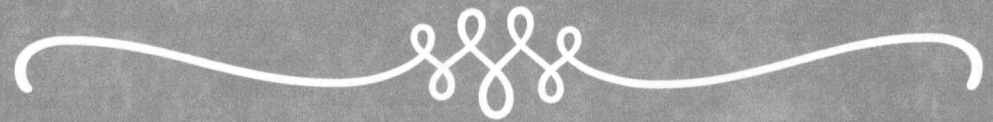

nutrition nugget
Mini Bites, Major Wins: Perfect for after-school snacks, movie nights, or anytime munching.

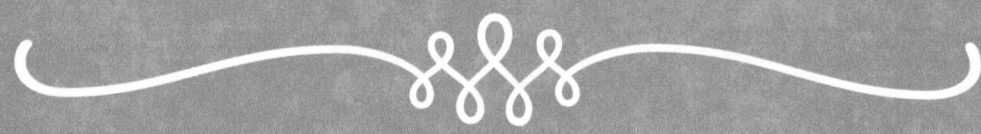

I truly believe that getting creative in the kitchen makes all the difference when it comes to feeding kids. Flavor, fun presentation, and hands-on cooking experiences can completely change how they view healthy food. That's why I love this recipe—it's packed with nutrients and turns snack time into a fun little adventure. Letting kids help out not only builds excitement but also makes them more likely to enjoy what they eat!

Zucchini pizza bites are the ultimate fun-sized snack—perfect as an appetizer or a healthy side dish. These mini bites are a creative way for kids to enjoy their veggies while still getting that classic pizza flavor they love!

Zucchini is loaded with vitamins, fiber, and antioxidants that support healthy growth and development. The small size makes them easy to handle (and less messy!), and the familiar combo of cheese and tomato sauce makes them more appealing to the kids. Plus, they are customizable, so you can add different veggies or protein to suit your child's taste! Use both white and yellow cheese for a colorful, melty effect that's extra tempting for kids.

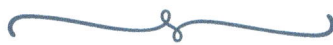

big pizza flavor, tiny veggie bite!

Why are these ingredients nutritious? Zucchini is a parent's best friend—mild in taste, packed with nutrients, and easy to sneak into just about any meal. Here's why it's a fantastic addition to a kid-friendly diet:

packed with goodness

Loaded with vitamin C, vitamin A, potassium, and fiber for growing bodies.

easy to digest

Its soft texture and high water content make it gentle on little tummies.

supports healthy vision

The beta-carotene in zucchini helps promote good eyesight, which is crucial for growing kids. Essential for screen time and homework!

great for hydration

With over 90% water, it helps keep kids refreshed and hydrated.

mild & versatile

ts mild taste makes it easy to sneak into meals—whether in muffins, pastas, or soups.

light but nutritious

Low in calories, high in nutrients—a win-win for little appetites.

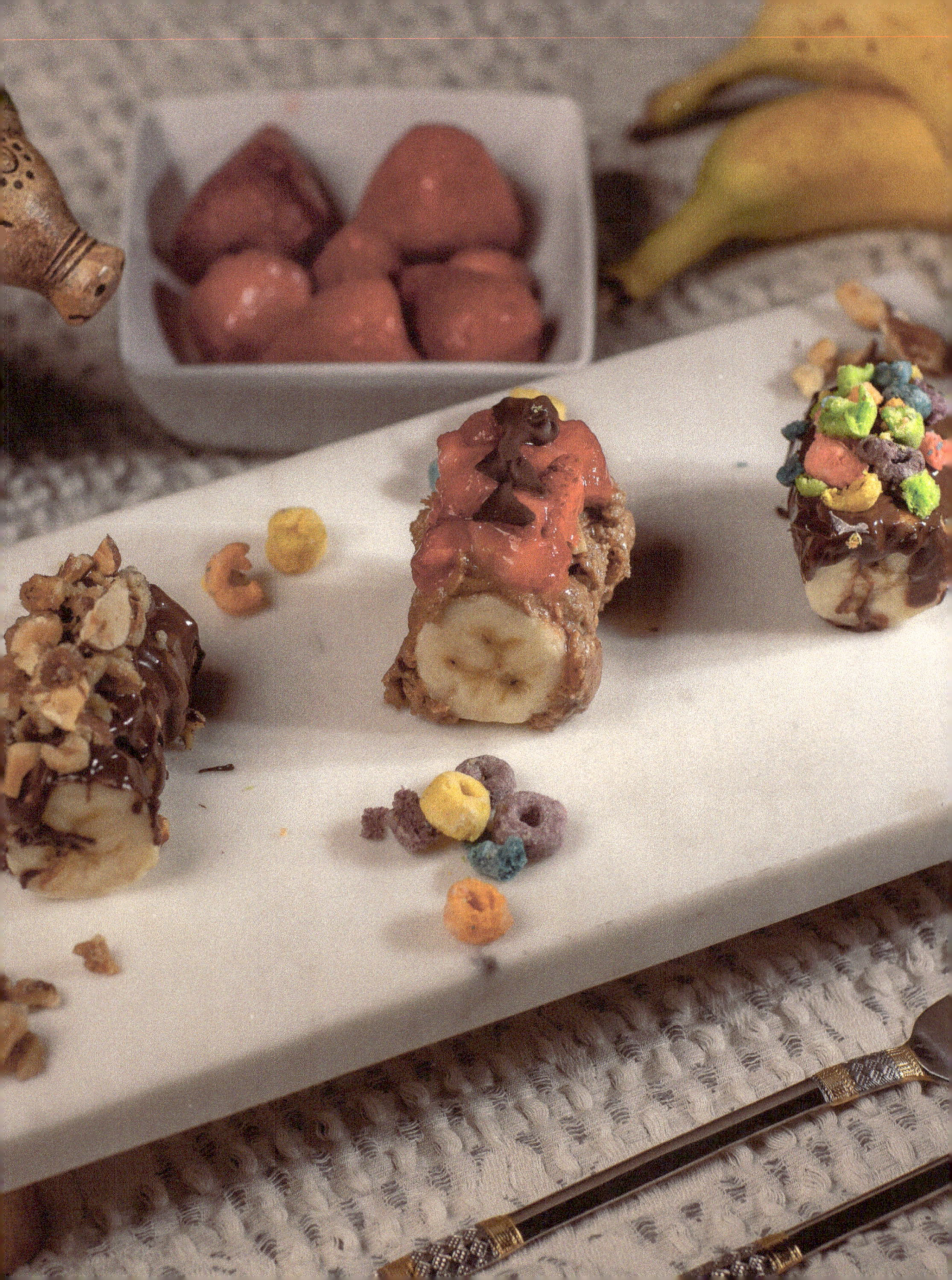

banana sushi

A fruity twist on sushi fun! In our home, the kitchen is more than a place to cook, where curiosity is celebrated and confidence is built, one fun bite at a time.

This banana sushi may be small, but it teaches kids that healthy food can be joyful, creative, and oh-so-rewarding.

Treat time just got a healthy upgrade! These simple, wholesome sweets are made to indulge, energize, and put a smile on your child's face without the sugar rush.

Packed with the natural sweetness of bananas and a fun twist, it's a creative, healthy treat that kids can enjoy making and eating together

banana sushi

Who knew a banana could be this much fun? Rolled up with love and packed with goodness! Banana sushi is a fun, nutritious, and creative after-school snack perfect for busy households! This playful fusion of tropical fruit and endless topping possibilities is sure to delight kids, even the pickiest eaters

ingredients

Topping 1
Peanut butter with fresh strawberries and chocolate chips
1 banana
1 cup fresh strawberries finely chopped
1/4 cup dark chocolate chips
3 tbsp peanut butter

Topping 2
Melted dark chocolate with crushed colorful cereal
1 banana
1/4 cup dark chocolate chips
1/2 cup crushed fruity cheerios cereal

Topping 3
Melted dark chocolate and jelly topped with granola
1 banana
5 tbsp crushed granola
1/4 cup dark chocolate chips
3 tbsp strawberry jelly

Topping 3
Melted chocolate with mixed nuts (almonds, walnuts, pecans, cashews)
1 banana
1/4 cup dark chocolate chips
4-5 tbsp crushed mixed nuts

directions

Peel the bananas and place them on a plate or board.

Peanut butter with fresh strawberries and chocolate chips
Spread the nut butter on top of the bananas. Sprinkle the bananas with chopped strawberries and chocolate chipsr

Melted dark chocolate with crushed colorful cereal
Melt the chocolate and pour it on top of the bananas. Place the cereal in a plastic bag and gently crush it using a rolling pin or a heavy-bottomed saucepan. Transfer the crushed cereal to a shallow bowl or plate. Roll the bananas in melted chocolate until evenly coated. Next, dip the coated bananas into the crushed cereal, ensuring they are well covered.

Melted dark chocolate and jelly topped with granola
Melt the chocolate and pour it on top of the bananas. Then layer it with jelly. Top the bananas with crushed granola.

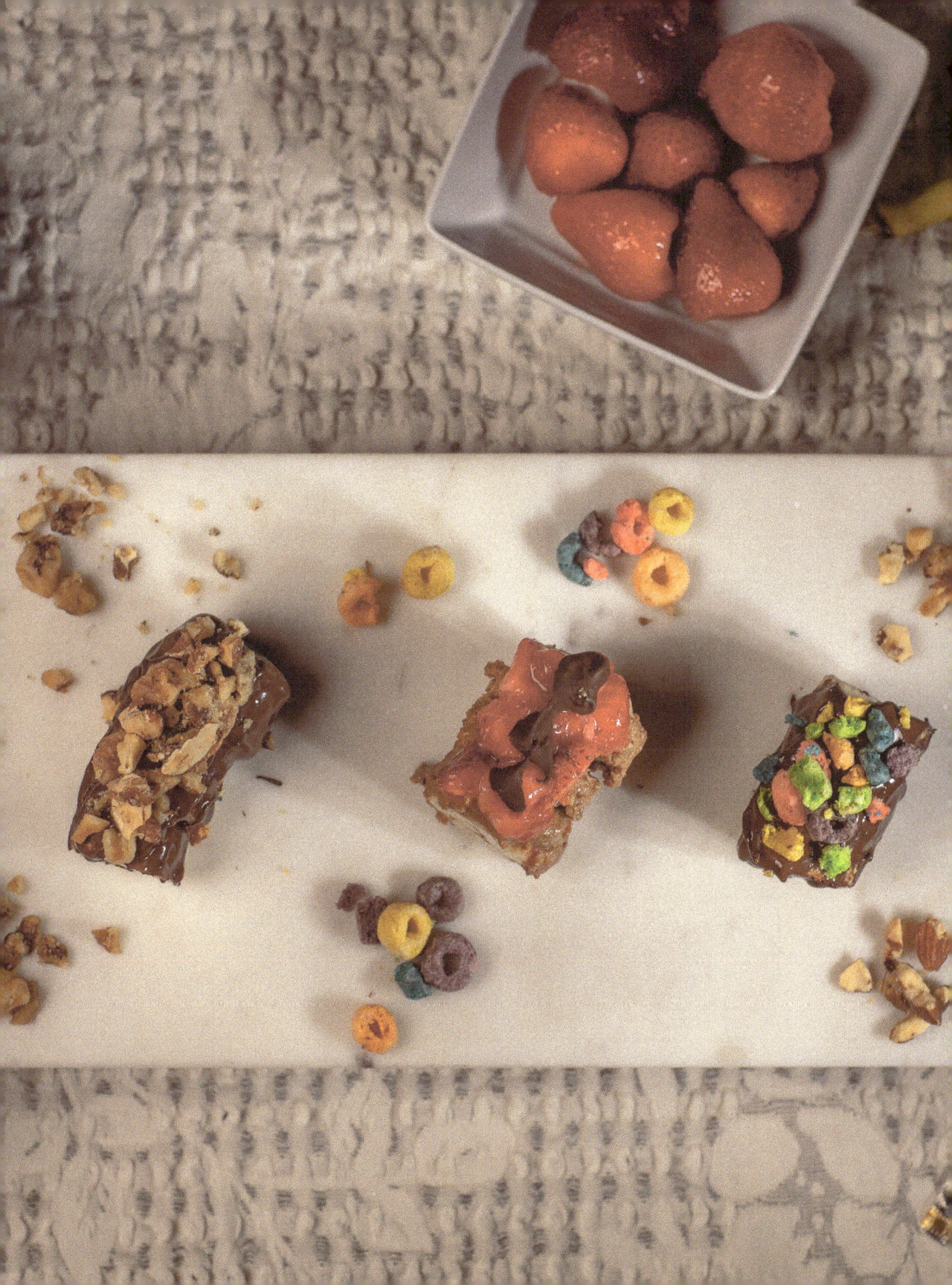

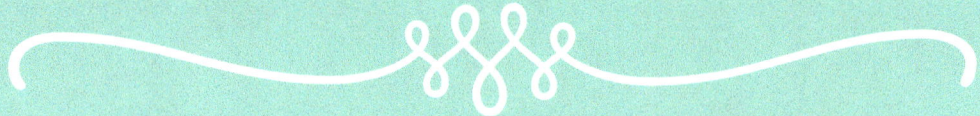

Banana sushi is a delicious and wholesome snack loaded with nutritional benefits.

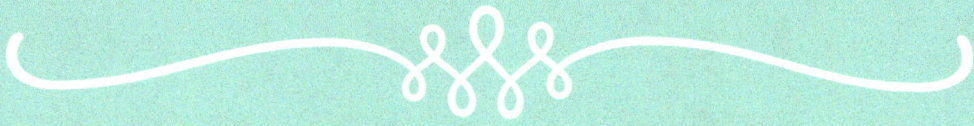

Melted chocolate with mixed nuts (almonds, walnuts, pecans, cashews)

Melt the chocolate and pour it on top of the bananas. Sprinkle the bananas with crushed mixed nuts.

Cut the bananas into bite-sized sushi pieces with a sharp knife.

Put them in the freezer for a couple of minutes, to allow the chocolate to set.

This banana sushi may be small, but it teaches kids that healthy food can be joyful, creative, and oh-so-rewarding.

fruit meets fun
healthy sushi kids can't resist

Banana sushi is a delicious and wholesome snack loaded with nutritional benefits. Let's dive into what makes it so great:

potassium powerhouse

Bananas bring heart-healthy potassium, vitamin B6, and digestion-friendly fiber to every bite.

energy on-the-go

Naturally sweet and energizing, bananas are perfect for keeping kids powered through playtime.

healthy fats & proteins

Toppings like peanut butter, almond butter, or Greek yogurt add protein and healthy fats for lasting fullness.

fiber fun

Rolling in crushed oats, whole-grain cereal, or chia seeds boosts fiber, aiding digestion and keeping kids full longer.

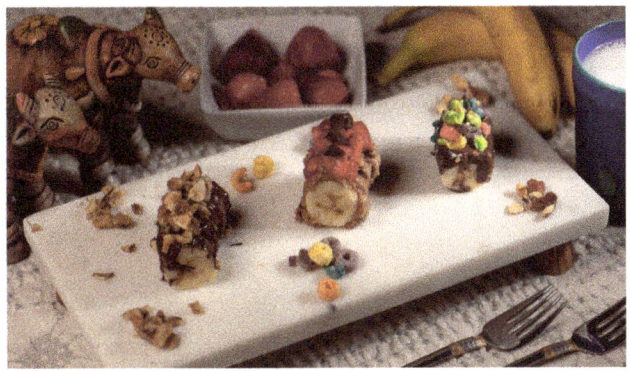

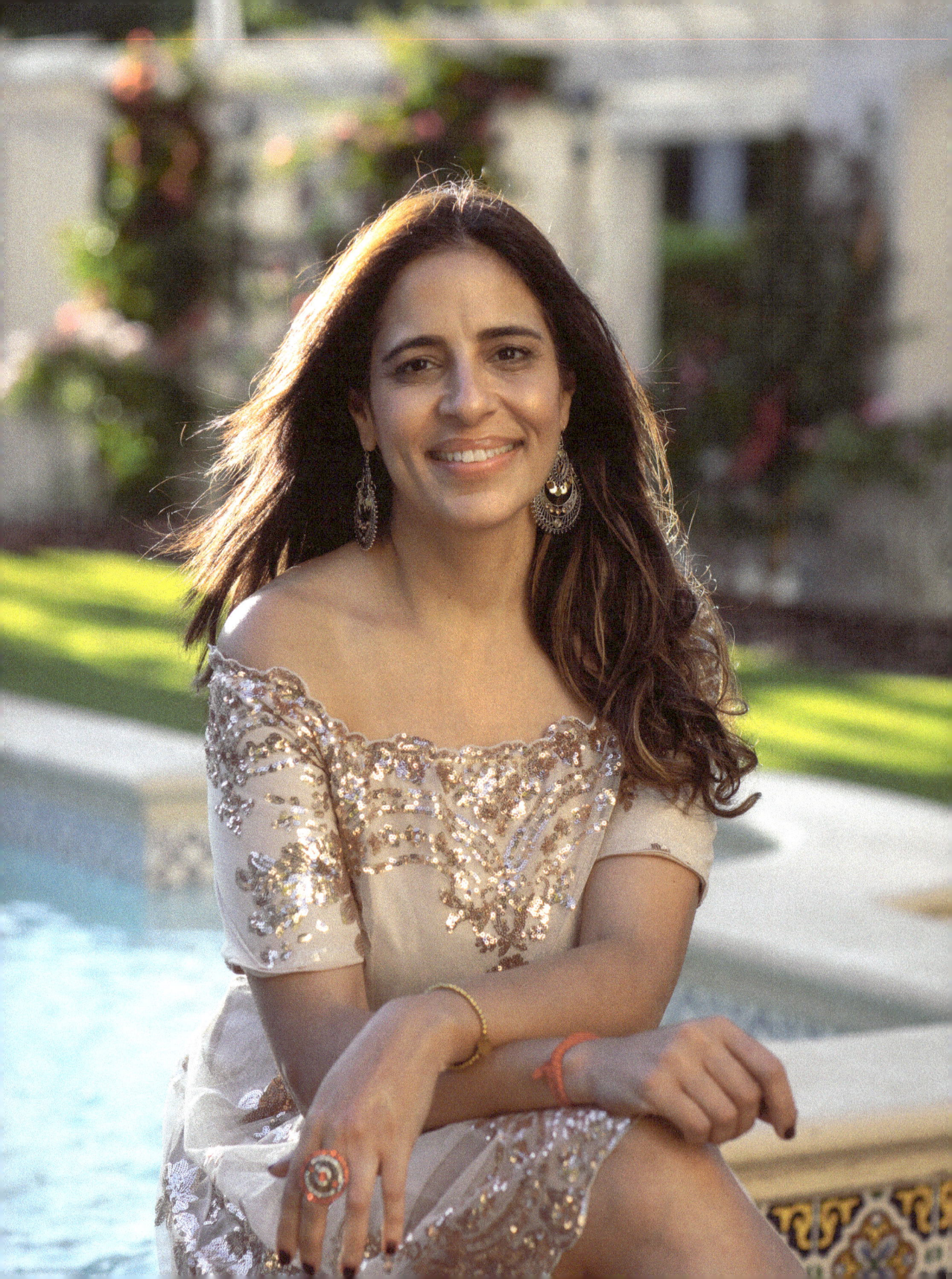